ROCKET TO THE MOON

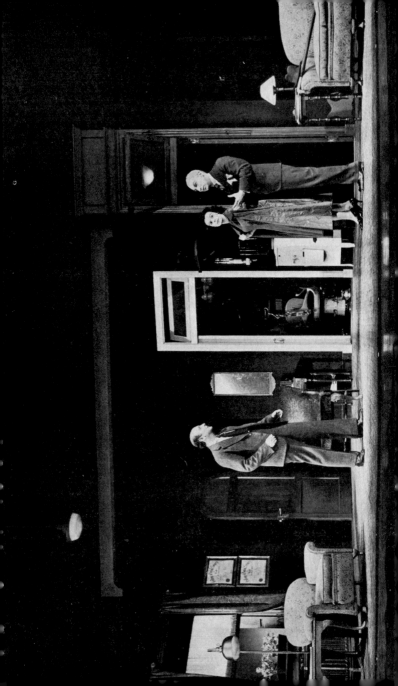

Rocket to the Moon

A ROMANCE IN THREE ACTS

BY CLIFFORD ODETS

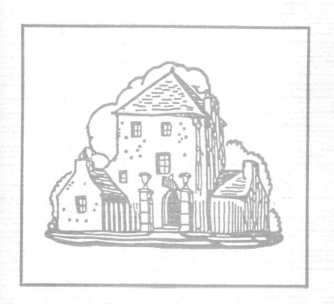

RANDOM HOUSE · NEW YORK

COPYRIGHT, 1939, BY CLIFFORD ODETS

FRONTISPIECE BY ALFREDO VALENTE

First Printing

MANUFACTURED IN THE UNITED STATES OF AMERICA

For Harold Clurman,
friend

Rocket to the Moon was first presented by the Group Theatre at the Belasco Theatre on the evening of November 24, 1938, with the following members of the Group Theatre Acting Company:

(In order of speech)

BEN STARK, D.D.S. . . . . MORRIS CARNOVSKY

BELLE STARK . . . . RUTH NELSON

CLEO SINGER . . . . ELEANOR LYNN

PHIL COOPER, D.D.S. . . . . ART SMITH

MR. PRINCE. . . . . LUTHER ADLER

FRENCHY . . . . LEIF ERICKSON

WILLY WAX . . . . SANFORD MEISNER

A SALESMAN . . . . WILLIAM CHALLEE

Directed by HAROLD CLURMAN
Settings by MORDECAI GORELIK

SCENES

ACT ONE

Dr. Stark's waiting room. A June afternoon.

ACT TWO

The same.

Scene I. An afternoon in July.
Scene II. Late afternoon, the beginning of August.

ACT THREE

The same. Night. The end of August.

ACT ONE

ROCKET TO THE MOON

ACT ONE

TIME: *The Present.*

PLACE: *A dentist's waiting room in a New York office building. A door to the elevators at the left. On the right side is a window. At the back are two doors, one leading to the dentist's office, the other open and showing the dentist's chair and apparatus. There is also a small hall, up right, which leads to another dentist's office.*

The curtain rises on the waiting room during an early hot June afternoon. Present are DR. BEN STARK *and his wife,* BELLE. *At the moment there is a strain and coolness between them, resulting from a family discussion on economics. In the silence* STARK *puffs strongly on his pipe as he looks at a page of a dental magazine in his hand.* BELLE *is depressed but hides it well.*

STARK

(*Finally*)

You've had your last word. There's nothing more to say.

BELLE

No, I want you to make up your own mind, or see that I'm right.

STARK

Aren't you always right, Belle?

BELLE

Ben, dear, such remarks are uncalled for.

STARK

You know I've wanted to specialize all my life. Yesterday your father proposes that I open a new office in a suitable neighborhood. He offers to bear all the expense, new equipment and all that. Look at that outfit—this x-ray unit! All night I didn't sleep thinking about it!

BELLE

Ben, you mustn't over-simplify—

STARK

(*Breaking in*)

Let's forget it, Belle.

BELLE

Poppa would pay the initial cost, but the rent there would be three times what it is here.

STARK

A little over two.

BELLE

A little less than three. You know the people here won't come uptown. It's too far away and that expensive neighborhood would frighten them off. It takes years to develop a practice. We had the experience twice—

STARK

(*Breaking in*)

You win, you win!

BELLE

(*Earnestly*)

It's not that I want to win, Ben. Don't you see that, Ben? Don't you see it?

STARK

(*Harshly, standing up*)

I told you let's forget it. It's settled! (*Moodily, after a pause*) I was a pioneer with Gladstone in orthodontia, once. Now I'm a dentist, good for sixty dollars a week, while men with half my brains and talents are making their twenty and thirty thousand a year!—I came over to the water cooler and I can't remember what for.

BELLE

To take a drink. . . .

STARK

I wanted to do something . . . what was it? Not a drink. . . . Oh, the flowers! (*He fills a paper cup, puts his pipe between his teeth and*

5

tries without success, one hand full, to fill a second cup.)

BELLE

Try one at a time, dear.

STARK

(*Coolly*)

One at a time is a good idea. (*At the window, right, he pours the water on a window box of drooping petunias. As he turns for more water he faces* BELLE *who has brought him the second cupful*) Thanks.

BELLE

(*Smiling*)

Any day now I'm expecting to have to powder and diaper you. (*Without an answer,* STARK *turns from the window and sits on the couch. After further silence, to make conversation:*)

STARK

I like flowers. . . .

BELLE

(*To ease the tension*)

You missed your profession, Ben.

STARK

(*Soberly*)

Botany?

6

BELLE

No, a florist shop.

STARK

I don't think you'd have married a florist.

BELLE

Why not? The way Poppa and Momma were always quarreling?—My nerves mincemeat? The way I felt when I married you, I'd have married a shoemaker almost.

STARK

I have a bunch of answers for that, but I won't give them.

BELLE

But he would have had to be calm and quiet, the way you were. You have such dignity, Ben . . . even when you're angry.

STARK

(*Annoyed*)

I'm not angry, dear.

BELLE

(*Softly*)

I know what it means to you. . . . (*Seductively*) Don't you think I know?

STARK

I know you know. . . .

BELLE

Tell Poppa what you decided. Is he coming here?

STARK

Some time this afternoon.

BELLE

Is it settled?

STARK

It's settled.

BELLE

(*Cautiously*)

Did Poppa bring up the question of moving in with us again?

STARK

Yes. . . .

BELLE

Don't encourage him.

STARK

(*Half indignantly*)

I don't, but I must say I can't understand how a father and daughter can be on the outs for so many years.

BELLE

If you'd seen the life of hell he gave my mother, you'd understand.

STARK

All right, but your mother's been dead a year. He's an old man, lonely—

BELLE

He'll manage—he's been to school.

STARK

I only mean that he's alone in the world—

BELLE

(*Seriously*)

A man and his wife should live alone, always. Poppa would be an intruder in our house. We wouldn't have a minute to ourselves. And out of sheer respect for my mother's memory—

STARK

Your father isn't a villain—

BELLE

Why do you take his part?

STARK

(*Again indignantly*)

I'm not, but after all, a man wants to spend

thousands of dollars putting me in a better practice and you expect me to think he's a villain?

BELLE

Now, Ben, you know he'd be in the way, don't
you?

STARK

(*Reluctantly, after a pause*)

I guess so. . . .

BELLE

Don't you know it?

STARK

(*With a faint ironic smile*)

Yes, mam. . . .

BELLE

(*Moving around the irony*)

Then it's settled.

STARK

(*Nodding his head*)

Umm.

BELLE

(*Crossing for purse*)

Where's the girl, your new secretary? My, my,
two hours for lunch—a fancy lady, indeed! That
girl isn't working out!

STARK

She's new at the job, dear. Give her time.

BELLE

She's taking plenty, two hours for lunch. And then the third week here you raise her salary. I don't understand you, Ben Stark.

STARK

Can a girl live on twelve dollars a week?

BELLE

I could manage if I had to, for the both of us.

STARK

Thank God we don't have to—

BELLE

It's not God who keeps us off the dole.

STARK

It's you, Belle. I don't know what I'd do without you! (*He puts his arms around her.*)

BELLE

Take the pipe out of my face. (*He moves his pipe and they kiss*) And now your terrible wife is going to give you another push. Did you put the ad in the paper? If we don't sublet the apartment soon, we'll have it on our hands all summer, and we can't afford it.

STARK

That's why Miss Singer's late. I asked her to put the ad in while she was out to lunch.

BELLE

She'll forget.

STARK

I'll eat my hat if she does. (DR. COOPER *enters from up right and crosses to the water cooler, where he drinks.*)

COOPER

Hot day.

BELLE

Yes.

COOPER

(Crossing back)

Beer makes you hotter. It's not a hot-weather drink like they think. (*Exits right again.*)

BELLE

(Lowering her voice)

I didn't know Dr. Cooper was in his office.

STARK

He's pouring some model or something. He's got his own troubles.

BELLE

How much does he owe us?

STARK

(*Sotto voce*)

Not so loud, Belle.

BELLE

(*Dropping her voice*)

How much?

STARK

(*Trying to remember*)

He hasn't paid his rent for three months.

BELLE

Four. Charity's a fine trait.

STARK

But it begins at home?

BELLE

You think it shouldn't? . . . Move the pipe away. Stop being soft-hearted. Will you be able to take a vacation this summer?

STARK

Why, we're taking a bungalow at the beach.

BELLE

That's a substitute for a vacation. Why can't we do what Jack and Milly Heitner do? Go to the

Rockies, or to Europe in the summer? But you're considerate of others. Not of yourself or your wife!

STARK

(*Slowly*)

I never thought of it that way.

BELLE

A woman wants to live *with* a man—not next to him. I see you three or four hours a night—in the morning you're gone before I get up. I'll elope some day. Then you'll cry your blue eyes black.

STARK

Every once in awhile I see something I didn't see before.

BELLE

What vision hit you now?

STARK

That being a dentist's wife is no joke—

BELLE

That's an old story—

STARK

(*With sudden buoyancy*)

I wish I could change everything. I'd buy Aladdin's lamp for a thousand dollars if I could. We'd

14

rub it up, we'd rub it down— Slam! We'd be in China—!

BELLE

I'll settle for Lake George— (*The door, left, opens. An elderly man walks in, quickly takes in the scene, and hastily exits.* BELLE's *back is to the door, but she catches* STARK's *glance*) Who was that?

STARK

Your father.

BELLE

Where?

STARK

(*Going to the door*)

He looked in and walked right out again.

BELLE

Don't call him. He'll be back in his own sweet time . . . in case you should both want to discuss me.

STARK

(*Surprised*)

Discuss you? Why?

BELLE

I heard him make a remark to you once: "The mother ate sour grapes and the daughter's teeth are set on edge." Ben, don't let poppa turn you

15

against me. Explain to him why you can't accept his offer—

STARK

Say, I see I've walked into something today.

BELLE

I happen to have been feeling blue all morning.

STARK

Why?

BELLE

Never mind. . . .

STARK

Tell me why.

BELLE

It doesn't matter, Ben . . . if you don't remember it.

STARK

What?

BELLE

Did you really forget, Ben? (STARK *is puzzled and tries to joke away her distressed look.*)

STARK

(*With a boyish twinkle*)

It's not your birthday and we were married in the winter. Or is it *my* birthday? . . . (*Then suddenly*) Oh . . .

BELLE

What?

STARK

You're thinking about . . . the boy?

BELLE

Yes. . . .

STARK

(*Putting his arms around her*)

Well . . . it's not as if we had him . . . he died at birth. . . .

BELLE

Three years ago this morning. I had him, I felt I had him. . . .

STARK

Don't think about it, dear.

BELLE

But never to be able to have another one . . . well . . .

STARK

Don't think about it, Belle.

BELLE

We could adopt a boy . . . if you wanted. . . .

STARK

Someone else's?

BELLE

If you wanted. . . .

STARK

We'll talk about it some other time, dear.

BELLE

Ben, you have to love me all the time. I have to know my husband's there, loving me and needing me.

STARK

(*Wanting to escape further involvement*)

Which I do, Belle, you know I do. Come on downstairs and let me buy you an ice cream soda.

BELLE

You know as much about women as the man in the moon!

STARK

I admit it. . . .

BELLE

No wonder your women patients don't like you.

STARK

They like me.

BELLE

Who? (CLEO SINGER *enters the waiting room.* STARK *quickly looks from secretary to wife and back again.*)

18

STARK

(*Sternly, for his wife's sake*)
You're late, Miss Singer—

CLEO

Late? Good afternoon, Mrs. Stark.

STARK

You're not supposed to take two hours for lunch.

CLEO

The buses take so long. . . . I'm sorry.

BELLE

Are you eating lunch in the Waldorf Astoria these days?

STARK

No, she went down to put the ad in.

CLEO

Ad? . . .

BELLE

(*Watching her closely*)
Eat your hat—she forgot it!

STARK

Did you?

CLEO

I meant to . . . Yes, it seems—

STARK

You're not very efficient, Miss Singer.

CLEO

It's so hot today.

BELLE

But how about the whole week? You had a whole week to clean the instruments and cut some cotton rolls for Dr. Stark.

CLEO

(*Helplessly*)

I'm going to do that right now, Mrs. Stark.

BELLE

No, right now you're going to take the ad to the *Times*.

STARK

(*To* BELLE)

She'd better stay here now. I'll send the ad down with a messenger boy. (*To* CLEO) You'd better change into your uniform.

CLEO

Right away, Dr. Stark. (CLEO *escapes into the office and closes the door behind her.*)

STARK

(*In a low voice*)

Let's not discuss her now.

BELLE

She has to be told—

STARK

Not now, Belle, not in front of her.

BELLE

Why not?

STARK

Belle, don't you think the girl has feelings? You and I are going downstairs. A soda for you, pipe tobacco for me. (*Seeing her face*) What's the matter, Belle?

BELLE

Go without me. I want to talk to her a minute.

STARK

Belle . . .

BELLE

On your way, Dr. Stark. (*He looks at her, shrugs his shoulders and starts for the door*) Put your street jacket on—be professional, Ben. (STARK *changes his dentist's gown for a street jacket, looks at his wife again and exits left. Clearing her voice and then calling)* Miss Singer!

CLEO

(Within)

Yes?

BELLE

Are you changing?

CLEO

Yes.

BELLE

I want to have a few words with you.

CLEO

(Opening the door but standing behind it)
I'll be out in just a sec', Mrs. Stark.

BELLE

You're dressed to kill, Miss Singer.

CLEO

That's one of my ordinary everyday dresses—angel-skin satin.

BELLE

It looks hot.

CLEO

(Coming into the waiting room in her uniform)
It's one of my coolest dresses.

BELLE

Is that why you don't wear stockings?

CLEO

Yes.

BELLE

(*Disapprovingly*)

I thought maybe to save money.

CLEO

I come from a well-to-do family.

BELLE

How well to do?

CLEO

I really don't need this job.

BELLE

(*Archly*)

Nevertheless, as long as you have the job, you should wear stockings in the office.

CLEO

Yes?

BELLE

Yes, it looks sloppy and it makes a very bad impression on the patients. Why do you wear your hair up in the air like that?

CLEO

Don't you like it this way?

BELLE

You're not modeling dresses now, Miss Singer.

CLEO

Oh, did Dr. Stark tell you—

BELLE

Dr. Stark tells me everything. The bills have to be sent out.

CLEO

I know that.

BELLE

Also, the reminder cards—

CLEO

I know that.

BELLE

(*Overly patient*)

If you know so much, why don't you do it?

CLEO

(*Flustered*)

You see, I was . . . (DR. COOPER *enters again from his office off right. He is wearing the usual dentist's gown. He is a big man, hot and troubled*

*at present. He speaks and moves in irregular un-
expected rhythms, but his manner is always frank
and winning. He is boyish and uncomplex, but
worried.*)

COOPER

Did the phone ring just now? Did I hear a
phone ring?

BELLE

No, you didn't, Dr. Cooper.

COOPER

I must be imagining things. (*Goes to water
cooler to drink.*)

CLEO

Probably.

COOPER

What?

CLEO

(*Innocently*)

I said probably. (*Seeing* BELLE *give her a strong
look*) I'll start on the bills now. (*She exits into
the office, closing the door behind her.*)

COOPER

(*Drinking*)

Municipal champagne! (*Sitting heavily*) Bills!
—She thinks people pay bills! I'm expecting a call.
What did you say?

BELLE

Nothing. . . .

COOPER

I'm hot—hot hot hot! In my younger days I was inclined to poetry. In my older days I'm inclined to poverty.

BELLE

What are your plans for the summer?

COOPER

What are the plans of a horse?

BELLE

You sound discouraged.

COOPER

My boy fell on his skates yesterday and broke his arm.

BELLE

I'm sorry to hear that.

COOPER

And that's the only break I've had in years! Yes, I went through the whole war and nothing happened to me. They could have left me there—

BELLE

You . . . owe us a few months' rent here.

COOPER

You have my sympathies.

BELLE

I know it's a bad time to remind you—

COOPER

To tell the truth, I'm waiting for a call from the loan company. I'll see what they have to say.

BELLE

(*Not unkindly*)

Why do you drink so much?

COOPER

Who drinks so much?

BELLE

Maybe it's coffee I smell.

COOPER

Yeah, Scotch coffee.

BELLE

Fair is fair, and if you share an office with another dentist, you have to share expenses. You won't do that by letting patients smell liquor on your breath, will you?

27

COOPER

What're you doing? Bawling me out?

BELLE

I'm telling you what I think.

COOPER

Maybe I'm not interested.

BELLE

My husband lets people walk all over him— Don't you think you're taking advantage of his good nature?

COOPER

That's a real nervy remark!

BELLE

(*Quietly*)

You don't meet your obligations.

COOPER

Sure, but give a man a chance!

BELLE

Dr. Cooper, to drink his practice away?

COOPER

(*Wrathfully*)

Who're you talking to? I'm not some shyster, some drunken bum!

BELLE

(*Patient, as with a child*)

Please don't shout.

COOPER

Is that what I am? A bum? Is that how I look to you?

BELLE

Nothing of the sort—

COOPER

(*After a pause*)

I don't blame you.

BELLE

For what?

COOPER

(*Sitting again*)

For looking out for your husband's interests. A civilized person can't tolerate me. Business won't pick up till after Labor Day. But if the loan company decides to— (*Within the office the telephone rings.* COOPER *quickly opens the door and takes the telephone from* CLEO's *hands*) Hello? . . . Yes, this is your party . . . yes . . . yes . . . yes . . . (COOPER *hangs up the telephone and trails back into the waiting room.* BELLE *sees* CLEO *staring out with curiosity and closes the office door on her*) No, no dice . . . no shoes for baby.

29

. . . I don't know what I'll do with my boy—
Children are not like furniture— You can't put
them in storage. If his mother was alive . . .

BELLE

(*Genuinely touched by his abject attitude*)
Stay another month. . . .

COOPER

(*Slowly*)

The summer'll be dead. Excuse me for the rum-
pus before. When I'm happy I'm a different person. You'd be surprised—everybody likes Phil
Cooper. (*He moves to the outer door, left.*)

BELLE

Where are you going?

COOPER

For a drink of coffee, Scotch coffee. (COOPER
exits. BELLE *goes to the side table for her purse
and gloves. From there she reaches up to the electric fan and slows it down a notch. Then she calls
to* CLEO.)

BELLE

Miss Singer?

CLEO

(*Opening the office door*)

Yes, Mrs. Stark?

BELLE

I'm going now. Tell Dr. Stark his terrible wife expects him home at seven. Good-bye.

CLEO

Good-bye. (*In crossing the room* BELLE *picks up the dental magazine which* STARK *left on the couch.*)

BELLE

Oh, one more thing. (*Handing over the magazine*) Put this in the office, like a good girl.

CLEO

Surely.

BELLE

Good-bye. (*As she looks* CLEO *over.*)

CLEO

Good-bye, Mrs. Stark. (*As* BELLE *goes to the door it is opened from the outside.* MR. PRINCE, BELLE's *father, enters again. He is near sixty, wears an old panama hat, a fine Palm Beach suit of twenty years ago and a malacca cane. There is about him the dignity and elegant portliness of a Jewish actor, a sort of aristocratic air. He is an extremely self-confident man with a strong sense of humor which, however, is often veiled. He is very alive in the eyes and mouth, the rest of him relaxed and heavy.* BELLE *looks at her father, who*

31

looks back at her with the same silence. He holds the door open for her as she exits. MR. PRINCE *slowly crosses and seats himself, leaning on his cane with both hands.)*

PRINCE
(With genuine curiosity)
Who are you?

CLEO
(Timidly)
Who are you?

PRINCE
(Pointing to the door)
I am the old father of that lady, so called.

CLEO
Mr. Prince?

PRINCE
(With suave gravity)
Yes.

CLEO
I heard of you.

PRINCE
From who?

CLEO
Frenchy.

PRINCE
Who?

32

CLEO

Frenchy—Dr. Jensen.

PRINCE

(*Moving restlessly around the room*)
You mean the foot doctor down the hall.

CLEO

Yes. Don't you speak to her?

PRINCE

No.

CLEO

Why?

PRINCE

(*Grandly*)

I am the American King Lear. (*Seeing her bewildered look*) Where is Dr. Stark?

CLEO

He'll be back in a minute.

PRINCE

And who are you?

CLEO

I'm the new secretary.

33

PRINCE

Hmm . . . what are your opinions?

CLEO

On what?

PRINCE

On anything. (*Taking newspaper from side table*) Here's the paper. Do you read? What are you? A communist? A fascist? A democrat?

CLEO

I don't know about all these things.

PRINCE

(*Glancing at the paper*)

Here it says in India a snake swallowed a man. What is your opinion of that, Miss . . . ?

CLEO

Singer.

PRINCE

What is that book in your hand?

CLEO

A dental magazine.

PRINCE

Leave it here—I like to look at pictures. (CLEO *gives him the magazine*) Are you afraid of me?

34

CLEO

No. . . .

PRINCE

Then why do you act nervous before me?

CLEO

I'm not nervous.

PRINCE

What's your first name?

CLEO

Cleo. . . .

PRINCE

Yes, Miss Cleo. . . . That's a name for a dancer. Do you dance?

CLEO

Yes.

PRINCE

You don't say!

CLEO

I've been with several shows.

PRINCE

You don't say! A dancer? What is the secret of life? Do you know?

CLEO

The secret?

35

PRINCE

I don't chew my cabbage twice, Miss Cleo. Let us pass on to my opinion of this (*Indicating the newspaper*) front page. Are you listening?

CLEO

Yes.

PRINCE

In my opinion the universe is governed by a committee; one Man couldn't make so many mistakes. (*Seeing* CLEO *laugh heartily*) Is that funny?

CLEO

Yes.

PRINCE

(*Smiling*)

I like to make people laugh. My daughter calls me a clown. The two of them, my wife included —with their bills they ate holes in me like Swiss cheese, but I was a clown!

CLEO

Mrs. Stark is very observant.

PRINCE

She annoys you?

CLEO

(*Withdrawing*)

I wouldn't say that.

36

PRINCE

Speak freely, Miss Cleo—

CLEO

Excuse me for being so personal before.

PRINCE

Everything that's healthy is personal.

CLEO

You're a very peculiar man, Mr. Prince.

PRINCE

Because I joke?

CLEO

Are you joking?

PRINCE

(*Twisting his hand from the wrist*)

Yes and no, hot and cold, like a shower. Do you have a gospel?

CLEO

(*Warily puzzled*)

What?

PRINCE

Every woman wants to convert a man to the gospel of herself. Fact? Fact! What is your gospel?

37

CLEO

(*After a pause*)

I don't understand a word you're saying, Mr. Prince!

PRINCE

It doesn't matter— I'm only a minor person in life. But I see you're honest.

CLEO

(*Narrowly*)

You're making fun of me!

PRINCE

(*Raising a hand*)

God forbid! You know something? . . . often I wished I was a young girl. I'd get somebody to support me—no worries about money—

CLEO

(*Flashingly*)

Nobody supports me!

PRINCE

A beautiful girl like you? Nobody supports you?

CLEO

No!

PRINCE

My remark makes you angry?

CLEO

Yes! I come from a very good home—

PRINCE

Miss Cleo, I think you need a revision of your philosophy—

CLEO

I heard enough from you! In fact I heard enough all day! I don't need this job. They burn your ears off around here for sixteen dollars a week. That's chicken feed!

PRINCE

(*More than agreeing*)

Less! *Pigeon* feed!

CLEO

(*Excited beyond diplomacy*)

I don't have to stand in Macy's window and let people throw rocks at me!

PRINCE

(*Calmly agreeing*)

Of course not.

CLEO

Am I the kind of girl who lets anybody make suggestive remarks to her?

PRINCE

No!

CLEO

Your daughter thinks—

PRINCE

Refer to her in the impersonal.

CLEO

Mrs. Stark, she thinks I'm a dummy. Do this, do that!—I'm a person!

PRINCE

One of the nicest I met in many years. Yes, Miss Cleo—

CLEO

And you?—You're an old fool!

PRINCE

(*Piously*)

What is age? A matter of psychology. Am I decrepit in my psychology?

CLEO

(*Tossing her head*)

I can't say!

PRINCE

The answer is no.

CLEO

And I don't care! If nobody cares for me I don't care for them!

PRINCE

Fair enough.

CLEO

I thought Dr. Stark was a nice man when I came here. But his wife just twists him around her little finger, like a spit curl.

PRINCE

Correct! And any woman could do the same.

CLEO

He stands there like a big shepherd dog and she tells him what to do!

PRINCE

Correct!

CLEO

He's afraid of his own shadow!

41

PRINCE

Correct!

CLEO

(*Excitedly*)

You can't get in my good graces by agreeing with me in everything I say. I see right through you, Mr. Prince, like cellophane.

PRINCE

(*Calmly*)

And when you look through the cellophane, what do you see?

CLEO

Never mind! How dare you say I have no opinions!

PRINCE

Did I say that?

CLEO

You insinuated that I was stupid—

PRINCE

Miss Cleo, I feel I know you for a lifetime.

CLEO

(*Scornfully*)

Thanks for the compliment!

PRINCE

You know something? You're just like me—

42

CLEO

Oh, no I'm not!

PRINCE

So you're not. Then who are you like?

CLEO

Like myself, like Cleo Singer! And I'm good and mad!

PRINCE

(*Suddenly snapping out*)

Calm down!

CLEO

What?

PRINCE

(*Sharply*)

Calm down. You have expressed yourself enough! You work here in an office—a regular insect society—so don't act like a tiger. Unless you don't want the job.

CLEO

(*Immediately contrite*)

Did I raise my voice?

PRINCE

(*Calmly*)

You don't know the facts of life, Miss Cleo.

43

CLEO

I'm not thinking of the job, but I'm sorry I hurt your feelings. Please excuse me.

PRINCE

Always address your elders with respect. They could leave you a fortune.

CLEO

I didn't mean to say all those things—

PRINCE

Do you get along well with people?

CLEO

No.

PRINCE

Why?

CLEO

(*Changing her mind*)

I get along with them.

PRINCE

Which is it?

CLEO

(*Distressed*)

I'm sorry I said so much. . . .

PRINCE

Are you going to cry, Miss Cleo?

CLEO

No.

PRINCE

I see dewdrops. . . .

CLEO

Something's in my eye.

PRINCE

(*Drawing a white silk handkerchief from breast pocket*)

Where? Which one?

CLEO

This.

PRINCE

Take your finger away. Look up. I won't hurt you. (*Delicately working on the eye*) Don't move. . . . (*Unseen by them* DR. STARK *opens the door. He watches the scene with disapproval.*)

PRINCE

Is it out?

CLEO

(*Blinking*)

I . . . think so.

45

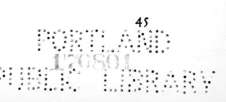

PRINCE

(*Standing off a little*)

Don't rub it.

CLEO

(*Blinking*)

No.

PRINCE

You use nice toilet water. It smells like thousands of flowers—

CLEO

Gardenia.

PRINCE

Pleasant.

CLEO

Forty dollars an ounce.

PRINCE

Unpleasant.

CLEO

That's a beautiful handkerchief.

PRINCE

You like it? Have it.

CLEO

Oh, no—

46

PRINCE

(*Spying* STARK)

Here is Benny, the shepherd dog. (CLEO *whirls around, guilt written all over her.*)

STARK

Hello, Poppa. . . .

CLEO

(*Rapidly*)

There was something in my eye and Mr. Prince—

STARK

Is it out now?

CLEO

It was nothing—

PRINCE

A glass splinter . . . from my daughter's heart.

STARK

(*With a slight frown, to* CLEO)

I think you'd better take that ad down to the *Times*, Miss Singer. Just slip your coat on . . . (*In the silence* CLEO *takes her coat and goes to the door, left.*)

CLEO

(*Lamely*)

Mrs. Stark says she expects you home at seven o'clock. She told me to tell you. . . . (*She exits.*)

STARK

(*Lightly*)

What was going on here?

PRINCE

(*Sitting*)

Just like she told you. (STARK *is changing jackets.*)

STARK

You're a great hand with the girls, Poppa.

PRINCE

It's the last thing in my mind.

STARK

But you mustn't talk that way about Belle in front of strangers.

PRINCE

Bad taste?

STARK

It doesn't happen to be true.

PRINCE

How old is Miss Cleo?

STARK

(*Smiling*)

None of your business. Where did you disappear to before?

PRINCE

(*Sauntering to the window*)

I often meant to ask you— What is that over there?

STARK

The back of the Hotel Algiers.

PRINCE

Hmm, I know a bookie in there. What must go on in those rooms at night . . .

STARK

What does it matter?

PRINCE

You got a decrepit psychology, Benny. Sometimes you talk like an old lady. (*Going back to his seat*) Do they rent out rooms to couples?

STARK

Riffraff.

PRINCE

Some night I'll come and look . . . just as if it interests me!

STARK

Tell me, what interests you, Poppa?

PRINCE

I love to gamble; cards, the races, the market . . .

STARK

Wine, women and song.

PRINCE

In all my life I never took a drink, and I don't sing. Yes, Benny, *I* started from an idealist, too, believe it or not. Now I'm a villain. . . . What does your friend Shakespeare say on this point?

STARK

What point?

PRINCE

The point of all points—happiness! Where is she hiding, happiness? (*After giving* STARK *a quizzical glance*) So when do you expect to move?

STARK

(*Nervously*)

Move?

PRINCE

(*Picking up the dental magazine*)

I see you turned down the pages—the machinery—

STARK

That Ritter outfit is a beauty. . . .

PRINCE

(*Seeing the other's hesitation*)

But?

STARK

I've decided to stay here for the present, Poppa. Not that your kindness—

PRINCE

Why?

STARK

Belle thought . . . she thinks it won't be wise.

PRINCE

(*Pursing his lips*)

I see. And you, what do you think?

STARK

After all, it's an economic risk. . . . (*He flushes off into silence.*)

PRINCE

(*Almost vehemently*)

Crazy boy, I offer it to you on a silver platter—

STARK

(*Painfully*)

That's how it is, Poppa.

PRINCE

Your nose is just the right shape to fit your wife's hand!

STARK

Is that a right thing to say?

PRINCE

Well, it's your life—yours and Mrs. Belle Stark!

STARK

Why do you insist, Poppa?

PRINCE

Because I like to do some good to a man who needs it! A lovable being!

STARK

Why don't you make it up with Belle?

PRINCE
(*With a smile*)

How's business?

STARK
(*Smiling*)

Slow. . . .

PRINCE

The summer slump?

STARK

Yes. Why don't you get along with Belle, Poppa?

PRINCE

(*Wryly*)

It's a pleasant June afternoon, Benny.

STARK

It grieves her very much.

PRINCE

(*Reluctantly*)

Benny, my daughter don't like me; she claims I ruined her mother's life. I claim her mother ruined *my* life!

STARK

How?

PRINCE

There are two kinds of marriages, Benny— where the husband quotes the wife, or where the wife quotes the husband. Fact? Fact!

STARK

But you didn't speak to her for ten years.

PRINCE

Because she insulted my soul, me, a first-class man, a lover of his brother man—

STARK

And his sister!

PRINCE

Never! *But never!* Not once did I make a sexual deviation! And what did I ask from my wife? To be a companion, to help me succeed—

STARK

You did—you're worth a fortune.

PRINCE

In spite of her! I shouldn't be ambitious. Go work for somebody else for twenty dollars a week —a man with my brains! Play safe! A housewife's conception of life! In the bargain, she had more respectability under the blankets than you have on Fifth Avenue! A man of my strength, my fire! (*Now masking his feelings again*) Drip, drip, the matrimonial waters go, and a man wears away. My wife is dead, I'm an old man who missed his boat. Ida Prince had her revenge . . . her husband has disappeared in the corner, with the dust, under the rug.

STARK

(*Grinning*)

Nonsense! You haven't disappeared, Poppa. You're a very dominant person—

PRINCE

(*Passionately*)

Without marriage I would have been one of the greatest actors in the world! . . . You don't believe it?

STARK

(*Having heard this before*)

I believe it. . . .

PRINCE

(*Suddenly*)

All my life I wanted to do something. . . . Pfu! . . . We'll talk of something pleasant.

STARK

After all is said and done, Poppa, Belle is your only child.

PRINCE

I'm her only father.

STARK

She's very lonely since Momma died. I feel sure she wants to bury the axe.

PRINCE

(*Cynically*)

Certainly. . . . Right in my head! I have a certain respectable mania for the truth—we don't like each other.

STARK

And yet you want to live with us.

PRINCE

You I like, Benny. But in my whole life one sensible woman came to my attention—she killed herself. She left a note, "I am a pest."

STARK

(*Shaking his head*)

You're in a bad mood today. . . .

PRINCE

(*Mopping his brow with the silk handkerchief and looking out at the Hotel Algiers again*)

True, true— (*Turning back from the window*) I made six thousand dollars this morning.

STARK

! ? !

PRINCE

The more money I make, the more heartache. Who'll I leave all my money to? Mrs. Belle Stark, née Prince?

STARK

(*Smiling*)

I know a certain orphan home in Philadelphia, where I was raised . . . they'd use it.

PRINCE

I don't know . . . maybe I'll leave it to Jascha Heifetz.

STARK

You going to Saratoga this summer?

PRINCE

Why should I drink Saratoga waters?—It only prolongs my life. (*Smiling slyly and winking*) Am I wrong? . . . Hotel Algiers. A man is a mirror. He tells me his wife is wonderful. . . . I look in his face to see the truth.

STARK

(*Uncomfortably*)

What do you see in my face?

PRINCE

A better liar than I gave you credit for. Is this the life you dreamed for yourself?

STARK

It's not Belle's fault.

PRINCE

One answer at a time. Is it?

STARK

(*Evasively, after a pause*)

I don't know what you mean. . . .

PRINCE

A life where every day is Monday. There used to be a week-end, but now it's always Monday. Awnings up, awnings down, coat on, coat off. Sweat in summer, freeze in winter—a movie, a bridge game, an auto ride to Peekskill. Gas is twenty cents a gallon, worry about the bills, write a budget—the maid is too expensive—you bought a pair of shoes *last* month. You're old, you're getting old—she's old. Yesterday you didn't look in my face. Tomorrow you forgot I'm here. Two aspirin pills are good for headaches. The world is getting . . . so dull, let me sleep, let me sleep! You sneeze, you have a cold. No, that was last month. No, it's now. Which is now and which is then? Benny . . . you used to be a clever boy! (*A silence follows, which* STARK *finally breaks.*)

STARK

(*Defiantly*)

Yes, a certain man once said that in our youth we collect materials to build a bridge to the moon; but in our old age, he says, we use the materials to build a shack.

PRINCE

(*Looking around the room*)

Yes, *this is it!* But you, you graduated first in the class! You played tennis, you were full of life and plans. Look, you don't even resent me now.

STARK

(*Slowly*)

I'm what I am . . . it's not Belle's fault!

PRINCE

What are you?

STARK

Not unhappy. . . .

PRINCE

You fell asleep at the switch. But Belle is worried—

STARK

Is she?

PRINCE

She's intelligent. You don't have children to hold you together. You're almost forty . . . a time for special adventures.

STARK

(*Stung, with sudden hotness*)

You have no right to speak this way! We're happy—

PRINCE

(*Cutting in*)

You're happy? You're sure of your future? You go home with a happy face at night?

STARK

Don't make trouble, Poppa!

PRINCE

(*Half smiling*)

Whose voice do you hear in your ear? Mine or yours? (*And then he smiles.*)

STARK

(*Slowing down*)

Gee, Poppa, I never know when you're serious.

PRINCE

A housewife rules your destiny. You love her?

STARK

Of course!

PRINCE

She's got you where she wants you. . . . Like an iceberg, three-quarters under water. . . . (*Pause*) I mightn't live forever. I want you to know what I think. (*He starts for the door.*)

STARK

You going home?

PRINCE

To my brokers and watch the board. My electric shares are going up. Your secretary uses too much paint and powder.

60

STARK

She'll tone it down.

PRINCE

(*Suddenly turning, hand on door knob, pointing his cane at* STARK *and lowering his voice to a near whisper*)

Iceberg, listen . . . why don't you come up and see the world, the sea gulls and the ships to Europe? (*Coming back into the room*) When did you look at another woman last? The year they put the buffalo nickel on the market? Why don't you suddenly ride away, an airplane, a boat! Take a rocket to the moon! Explode! What holds you back? You don't want to hurt Belle's feelings? You'll die soon enough—

STARK

I'll just have to laugh at that!

PRINCE

Laugh. . . . But make a motto for yourself: "Out of the coffin by Labor Day!" Have an affair with—with—with this girl . . . this Miss Cleo. She'll make you a living man again.

STARK

(*Laughing*)

You're a great joker, Poppa. (PRINCE *follows* STARK'S *laughter; both men laugh together.*)

PRINCE

. . . Never look away from a problem, Benny.

STARK

I never know when you're serious.

PRINCE

When you look away from the problem, it don't disappear. But maybe *you* might disappear! Remember I told you! (PRINCE *abruptly exits.* STARK *is still laughing; now he suddenly stops, mouth half open. He is not feeling humorous and he realizes it in a flash. Rather he is now depressed, even frightened a little. Twice he mutters to himself.*)

STARK

"Sonofagun! . . . Sonofagun! . . ." (*Now* DR. JENSEN, *a chiropodist with office down the hall, commonly called Frenchy, breezes into the waiting room. He is an American of Swedish parents, aged thirty, realistic and alert, fast and practical. He has an active wiry body; wears a white jacket. Now he pins the door back.*)

FRENCHY

Hello, Doc. Pin back the door—it's hot. (*Goes to water cooler.*)

STARK

(*Abstracted*)

Hello, Frenchy.

FRENCHY

Some day, when I can afford it, I'll get a water cooler. You don't mind me running in and out like that, do you? (*He sits.*)

STARK

(*Depressed*)

Of course not, Frenchy.

FRENCHY

The Palm Beach kid was here again.

STARK

Who?

FRENCHY

Mr. Prince. He gave me a gloomy hello in the hall.

STARK

He's a gloomy man.

FRENCHY

Why?

STARK

I can't make out. He disturbs me.

63

FRENCHY

Why?

STARK

Every time he drops in here I'm depressed for hours after.

FRENCHY

Make a phonograph record—let me listen.

STARK

You wouldn't understand. You have to be married first.

FRENCHY

I see.

STARK

Do you know something about women?

FRENCHY

What?

STARK

No, I mean do you know anything about women?

FRENCHY

I'll be explicit: no!

STARK

(*Musingly*)

A man falls asleep in marriage. And after a time he wants to keep on sleeping, undisturbed. I'm

surprised how little I've thought about it. Gee!—
What I don't know would fill a book.

FRENCHY

(*Watching him*)

You look like helplessness personified.

STARK

He tries to tell me I'm dissatisfied with my married life—

FRENCHY

Maybe you are. . . .

STARK

He's very persuasive in some things, but I know
he's incorrect. (*Suddenly grinning*) Do I look like
an unhappy man?

FRENCHY

(*After a pause, soberly*)

You'd know that better than me, Doc.

STARK

(*Shaking his head again*)

Sonofagun! . . . Don't all married couples
argue and disagree? Even the joke papers tell us
that. A man would be a mad idealist to want a
honeymoon all his life.

FRENCHY

No, he'd be a woman. A man can't be both lover and banker, enchanter and provider. But the girls want those combined talents. . . . The man who worries for the bucks is not the one to kiss his wife behind the ear.

STARK

Yes. . . . (*But continuing with his own thoughts*) There's something positively *sinister* about that man!

FRENCHY

Prince? *Cynical.*

STARK

I don't understand human nature, not the off-color things. Suddenly he tells me he wants to be an actor! I like normal people, like you.

FRENCHY

Hell, who's normal nowadays! Take that kid of yours, that Cleo—

STARK

Sometimes people embarrass me. The most ordinary people suddenly become sinister—

FRENCHY

Sinister? They're just sleepy.

STARK

What about Miss Singer? You were saying—
(COOPER *enters the waiting room, distracted and
brooding.*)

FRENCHY

(*With a glad shout*)

Here's Coop! Let's hear what he has to say.

COOPER

(*Sitting heavily*)

What?

FRENCHY

What's your opinion of women, Coop?

COOPER

Who's got time to think about women! I'm trying to make a living!

FRENCHY

(*Turning to* STARK *with a laugh*)

You see!

COOPER

Is there a man in our generation with time to
think about women? Show me that man and I'll
show you a loafer!— (*To* STARK) Did anybody
call me while I was out?

STARK

No.

COOPER

This morning I had a hunch there'd be some business. Nobody called?

STARK

No.

(*Notice here* FRENCHY'S *constant activity of watching people, listening and probing them, watching their reactions to things he says and does. It must be confessed: He is a self-educated, amateur student of human nature in all its aspects.*)

COOPER

(*After a pause*)

It's gonna be a hot summer. . . .

STARK

Nothing on your calendar today?

COOPER

(*With a snort*)

Yeah! At four o'clock a distant relative is coming in for a free cleaning. (*Mopping his brow*) I'm dead! (*Pause*) Your wife made me a proposition, to put up or get out.

STARK

When? !

COOPER

Recently. She almost chewed my head off. Before.

STARK

(*Embarrassed, trying to explain*)
She thinks people take advantage of me. . . .

FRENCHY

You're doing those W.P.A. boys' work for half price—that's advantage.

STARK

I hope she doesn't hear about it.

FRENCHY

It's her business to hear about it: every generous impulse on your part brings her closer to insecurity.

COOPER

(*Defensively, annoyed*)
You're a big busybody, Frenchy!

STARK

(*Protestingly*)
You can't let poor boys like that just walk out.

FRENCHY

I know plenty who let them walk.

COOPER

Walk yourself, please—I have to talk business here.

FRENCHY

(*Giving* COOPER *a shrewd look*)

Excusé moi. . . . I'll go back and take a nap.

STARK

In the middle of the day?

FRENCHY

(*Going to the door*)

Why not? Just had my lunch. A snake eats a rabbit and falls asleep, don't it? Why should I be better than a snake? (FRENCHY *laughs and exits left.*)

COOPER

He's a madman. (*An uncomfortable silence ensues*) Who wears the pants in your family, Stark?

STARK

(*Indignantly*)

Belle had no right to tell you that!

COOPER

(*Humble in the face of necessity*)

Tell her you decided to let me stay in the office till after Labor Day. How is that for a request?

(*After waiting for an answer*) She might object . . . ?

STARK

I'll decide that, Phil!

COOPER

Well, that's my problem in a nut shell. You'll have an empty office on your hands if I leave.

STARK

Where would you go?

COOPER

In the park and eat grass.

STARK

(*Shocked back to attention*)

As bad as that? (*After another uncomfortable pause*) Can't you pay anything, Phil?

COOPER

No. . . .

STARK

I mean . . . you know . . .

COOPER

Sure. . . .

STARK

(*Finally*)

. . . You'd better stay here till something happens. You can't move now.

COOPER

In July I'll pay a month—I'll get the money.

STARK

(*Uncomfortably*)

You know how it is. . . .

COOPER

So it's settled?

STARK

Yes.

COOPER

(*With the joy of relief*)

You gave me a new lease on life! You're good, you're kind, you're generous to the nth degree!

STARK

(*Embarrassed*)

No, I'm not. . . .

COOPER

Hail, Ben Stark!

72

STARK

Stop it, Phil. . . .

COOPER

No, I mean it, every word!

STARK

I hope things pick up for you.

COOPER

You're a pride to me, a pleasure! Now I'll go down for a shave. Again, thanks. (*He offers his hand, which* STARK *takes.*)

STARK

Shhh! (*With a laugh and a wave of his hand,* COOPER *starts for the exit, right.* CLEO SINGER *enters,* COOPER *almost knocking her down.*)

COOPER

Miss Singer, you're a lovely girl. Take any messages for me. (COOPER *exits, left.* CLEO *stands in her place a moment, surprised.* STARK *looks at her as if he had never seen her before, secretly examining her throughout the following scene. Because of his previous scene with* PRINCE *she now presents a challenge to him which he might never have come to alone.*)

CLEO

Why did he say that?

STARK

He's feeling good.

CLEO

(*Taking off her coat*)

I almost roasted to death in this coat. They call weather like this earthquake weather in California.

STARK

Were you ever there?

CLEO

Surely, several times. (*Hanging up the coat*) The more expensive kinds of camel hair don't wear well, do they?

STARK

Did you put the ad in?

CLEO

I don't forget my duties twice, Dr. Stark.

STARK

(*Appeased by her attractive humble air*)

I owe you an apology for the way I shouted at you before.

CLEO

(*Pleasantly*)

Into every life a little rain must fall. I don't mind.

74

STARK

(*Hesitantly*)

You'd be much more attractive . . . if . . . you didn't . . . use so much lipstick.

CLEO

Too much? . . . It's so dark at this mirror here. (*Goes to the wall mirror.*)

STARK

It's only my opinion, Cleo—

CLEO

(*Turning rapidly*)

Do you realize that's the first time you've called me Cleo since I've been here? !

STARK

(*Taken aback*)

Is there any reason why I shouldn't?

CLEO

Oh, no! Certainly not!

STARK

How old are you, Cleo?

CLEO

(*Coquetting slightly*)

Don't you think that's a personal question?

STARK

I have no personal motives. . . .

CLEO

(*Smiling back*)

Mr. Prince asked me the same thing. He's a terrible flirt, isn't he?

STARK

(*Frowning*)

That's his way. He tries to be interesting—

CLEO

Lots of men are trying to be interesting.

STARK

Are they?

CLEO

(*She starts for the office door but stops short*)

Would you mind if I don't wear stockings in the office in the summer? Mr. Bernstein at Chelsea-Pontiac didn't mind.

STARK

Well . . .

CLEO

(*Hastily*)

If you say not to—

STARK

(*Ditto*)

It's quite all right.

CLEO

Your wife might object.

STARK

Why should she?

CLEO

I may be wrong, but so many wives like to keep an eye on their husband's secretary.

STARK

Mrs. Stark runs my home. I run the office.

CLEO

After all, we must keep cool, mustn't we? May I say this?—I like you, Dr. Stark. Maybe that's too personal, but everything that's healthy is personal, don't you think?

STARK

(*Ponderously*)

Very possible. . . . (CLEO *stops at the side table on her way to the office again.*)

CLEO

Looking at this newspaper makes me think—the universe must be ruled by a committee; one man couldn't be so stupid.

STARK

(*Smiling*)

That's a very witty remark!

CLEO

(*Pleased*)

I'm glad you think so, Dr. Stark.

STARK

(*Looking at his watch*)

Mrs. Nelson will be here any minute. You'd better clean up the instruments, particularly the scalers.

CLEO

The scalers? . . . Which are those, Dr. Stark? I know, but I want to make sure.

STARK

(*Taking one from his top pocket*)

These.

CLEO

I'll cut some cotton rolls, too.

78

STARK

Always dry an instrument when you remove it from the sterilizer. It'll clean easier.

CLEO

That's a very good hint.

STARK
(*Dryly*)

I wasn't hinting. Patients like clean instruments.

CLEO

Of course. (*Stopping at the operating room door*) Your wife was very angry with me before.

STARK
(*Impatiently*)

Mrs. Stark is not the terrible person many people think she is!

CLEO
(*Dismayed*)

Oh, I didn't mean anything. . . .

STARK
(*Almost savagely*)

She's one of the most loyal, sincere and helpful persons I've ever met!

CLEO

(*In a small voice*)

I'm sure she is, I'm sure of that. . . . (CLEO *now disappears into the operating room. For a moment* STARK *stands there, wagging his head. His eye falls on the dental magazine. He picks it up, looks at the ad and then throws the magazine across the room. As he begins to fill his pipe his glance turns to the window, right. He moves over to the window and looks out at the Hotel Algiers.* CLEO's *voice from the operating room threshold turns him around with a guilty start. In a small contrite voice*) Pardon me . . . did I tell you before? Your wife expects you home at seven.

STARK

(*Annoyed*)

Yes, thanks—you told me—thanks!

CLEO

(*Meekly*)

You're welcome, Dr. Stark. (CLEO *disappears into the operating room again.* STARK *looks after her, annoyed. For a moment he stands reflectively. Finally he strikes a match and begins to light his pipe.*)

Slow Curtain

ACT TWO

ACT TWO

Scene I

PLACE: *The same.*
TIME: *July.*

DR. STARK *is standing where we last saw him, now perusing a small volume of Shakespeare and smoking his pipe. He is much calmer than when last seen.* FRENCHY *is lazily turning over the pages of a picture magazine, his attention obliquely on* CLEO. *She sits near the water cooler, hands in lap, frankly watching and examining* DR. STARK. *Above the electric fan hums busily; the outward door is held back for any possible extra ventilation.*

DR. STARK'S *pipe has gone out—he puffs on it strongly.* CLEO *immediately gives him a paper of matches. Then she crosses to the water cooler and drinks. Next she brings a cup of water to* STARK. FRENCHY *watches all of this.*

CLEO

I thought you'd like some cold water, Dr. Stark. It's so hot.

STARK

Thank you, Cleo.

CLEO

That's all right. . . . (*A quick glance passes between them,* FRENCHY *not missing it. To make conversation*) Is that Shakespeare which interests you so much?

STARK

(*Turning the book over in his hand*)

This? Yes, this is the very copy Dr. Gladstone gave me fifteen years ago. . . . Fifteen? Can that be right? . . . Yes, it's fifteen years ago. (*Shaking his head*) Gosh . . .

CLEO

Was he your teacher?

STARK

Yes, and he was best man at my wedding, too. Shakespeare's a companion, he said— Whatever you want to know, look in his plays.

CLEO

Like a Bible?

STARK

Like a Bible. It was a great loss to me when Dr. Gladstone died. A wonderful man. Mrs. Stark didn't like him—

FRENCHY

(*Suddenly*)

Must be hell to sleep two in a bed these nights.

STARK

(To FRENCHY)

What? Did you say something?

FRENCHY

The days and nights are just a congregation of sodden hours. (CLEO *seats herself and crosses her legs*) Yeah, July is a month for celibacy.

CLEO

What does that mean, celibacy?

FRENCHY

(Looking across at her)

Your skirt is up to your neck. (*After* CLEO *hastily adjusts her skirt*) Up at Fire Island yesterday a man collapsed from the heat while clipping a hedge. (CLEO *is and has been annoyed for days by* FRENCHY's *consistently insolent attitude toward her.*)

CLEO

Dr. Jensen, you may be the world to your mother, but you're no joy to us. We know it's hot—

FRENCHY

(Sharply)

Don't be so fresh, Angel Skin!

85

CLEO

(*Immediately cowed*)

I'm sorry. . . .

FRENCHY

You make me rue the day I picked you out of fifty-three girls for this job.

CLEO

(*Defiantly*)

It seems to me that Dr. Stark could have picked me just as well.

FRENCHY

Except that he was too shy to look them over. You pushed that jingling body in my face and you got the job. It was a moment of aberration for me.

STARK

(*Protestingly*)

Frenchy, what are you saying?

FRENCHY

It's the heat— Do I know what I'm saying?

CLEO

Some people say more than is good for them!

FRENCHY

(*Warningly*)

Some people *do* more!

CLEO

(*Indignantly*)

Sometimes you act as if you're talking to an animal!

FRENCHY

What's in a name? Look at me. They call me Frenchy. Why? Cause I'm a Swede. . . . A little Swede from Utica, New York.

CLEO

Well, I don't like it—you keep picking on me!

FRENCHY

(*Contemptuously*)

You gonna cry?

CLEO

(*Scoffingly*)

What for?

STARK

Frenchy likes you, Cleo.

CLEO

Yes, like poison! God knows why—I never did anything to him.

FRENCHY

(*Significantly*)

And don't do anything to my friends either.

STARK

(*Puzzled*)

What are you talking about?

CLEO

He wouldn't talk about me that way if my brother was here.

FRENCHY

What's your brother, a fireman or a cop?

STARK

(*To* CLEO)

Goodness, he's not talking about you.

CLEO

Well, he's looking me straight in the eye.

FRENCHY

(*Changing the subject*)

How is it you live down the beach and don't look sunburnt, Doc?

STARK

I spend only Sundays and an occasional Saturday in the sun.

FRENCHY

You must be coining money here.

STARK

My wife hasn't made a bank deposit in several weeks.

FRENCHY

I'm very satisfied to live on twenty-thirty bucks a week. They got me all steamed up in school about being president, but this suits me from the ground up.

CLEO

(*Scornfully*)

The ground *down*, you mean.

FRENCHY

(*After a glance, ignoring her*)

Fire Island's getting awful crowded though. Some show people moved up there last week.

CLEO

(*Immediately interested, coming forward*)

Show people? Who?

FRENCHY

(*Shrugging*)

I should worry who.

CLEO

From the legitimate?

FRENCHY

I should worry. (*Waving the magazine in his hands*) I sent a snapshot to this picture paper— "Dr. Walter Jensen—Frenchy to his friends— Manicuring Milady's Feet." But they didn't print it. No matter what you do, you can't make people foot-conscious. (FRENCHY *looks at a few more pictures. In the meantime* CLEO *has gone to the wall mirror. Looking into the mirror she lifts her damp hair from the back of her neck. She sees* STARK'S *eyes on her and offers the following explanation,* FRENCHY *observant and listening.*)

CLEO

You get so damp under here, right at the neck.

STARK

Why don't you keep it up?

CLEO

Keep the hair up? Mrs. Stark told me not to. . . .

STARK

When was that?

CLEO

Oh, weeks ago. She said I wasn't modeling dresses here.

STARK

(*After giving* FRENCHY *a quick look*)
She must have been joking.

CLEO

No, she said—

STARK

(*Quickly*)
You wear it any way you like, the most comfortable . . .

FRENCHY

(*Dryly, intent on the pictures*)
My, Doc, we're getting independent.

CLEO

(*Flashing a haughty look at* FRENCHY)
I'll do that, Dr. Stark.

FRENCHY

(*Rising from his seat*)
I'll return this paper after.

STARK

Okay.

FRENCHY

Maybe my office cooled off.

CLEO

(*Saucily*)

You oughta pay rent on two offices, Dr. Jensen.

FRENCHY

(*Scornfully*)

I'm not sure what's going on in your fertile brain, Juicy Fruit. . . . But you stripped your gears with me. (*He drifts out of the office. There is a momentary silence.*)

STARK

Don't mind him—he's peculiar.

CLEO

(*With lofty superiority*)

Don't worry, I don't. I take the source into account.

STARK

(*With sudden unrestrained eloquence*)

"For slander's mark was ever yet the fair;
The ornament of beauty is suspect,
A crow that flies in Heaven's sweetest air.
So thou be good, slander doth but approve
Thy worth the greater. . . ."

92

(*With apologetic embarrassment now*) Shakespeare. . . .

CLEO

Oh, that's nice. Shakespeare? Do you know something? I can't read Shakespeare—the type is too small.

STARK

That isn't all editions—

CLEO

(*Hastily*)

Oh, of course it isn't. I know it isn't—of course. (*After a pause*) Dr. Jensen don't seem to have any manners, does he? His personality is really nil, isn't it?

STARK

I wouldn't say that. . . .

CLEO

An interesting personality must have a foundation of good character.

STARK

Who told you that?

CLEO

No one has to tell me such things. Dr. Jensen really offends. He does not know and obey the fundamental rules of etiquette.

STARK

He's a self-educated man—

CLEO

That don't cut no ice— So am I. My parents wanted to send me to a fashionable girl's college, but I went to secretarial school instead—just for the experience. Notwithstanding, I know the correct things to do and say. My husband, when I get married, will find me the perfect hostess.

STARK

(*Not knowing what to say*)

Do you intend to marry?

CLEO

I don't know—marriage is so sordid. I'd never marry for money. (*Abruptly*) Do you love your wife?

STARK

(*Torn between her foolishness and attractiveness*)

Yes. . . .

CLEO

That was a ridiculous thing to ask, wasn't it?

STARK

No.

CLEO

She must be an ideal wife.

STARK

You think so?

CLEO

I've often admired her for the way she manages and takes care of herself.

STARK

Do you like her?

CLEO

She has very good manners. God knows, there's not much courtesy left in the world! . . . May I be frank, Dr. Stark?

STARK

Yes.

CLEO

I've often resented the way she speaks to you.

STARK

How?

CLEO

Perhaps I better not mention it. . . .

STARK

You can. . . .

CLEO

Well, she seems angry with you, Dr. Stark.

STARK

(*Half smiling*)

Isn't that permissible?

CLEO

Permanently? I may be wrong. . . .

STARK

That's just your impression.

CLEO

It must be. . . . (*Seeing him smile*) Everything amuses you, Dr. Stark.

STARK

(*Very close to her*)

Why?

CLEO

You're smiling.

STARK

It just seems that way. It's a habit. . . . When I can't meet a situation, I smile as if it amuses me. I don't mean to, but it comes out that way.

CLEO

Don't you feel foolish sometimes?

STARK

To tell the truth, yes. . . .

96

CLEO

I think you're not a happy man. You have so much to live for—I can't see why. Have you got troubles?

STARK

No.

CLEO

Do you mind my saying this?

STARK

No.

CLEO

I think happiness is everything. You can have a castle, and what have you got if you're not happy? An important person once told me Mr. Rockerfeller—you know, that one, his father—he had a silver windpipe. With all that money! It goes to show you.

STARK

True. . . . Are you?—Happy?

CLEO

Oh, yes! Life is so full of a number of things! Parties, dances— But I do resent having to change so often—

STARK

Change?

CLEO

You know, clothes—it irks me. Cruises are pleasant. I've taken several of those, but not recently. A girl makes a mistake to go alone on a cruise; it makes you so conspicuous.

STARK

(*Quietly, but completely aware of her*)

Life must be very pleasant for you.

CLEO

Yes, it is. That's why I didn't mind in the least when you said we'd have to work late tonight. Most of my friends are away for the summer— the city's dead. (*After a pause*) Summer is beautiful, I think. All the people have such an unbuttoned mood, don't they? People can be so kind and good when they're relaxed, can't they?

STARK

(*Touched by her genuine lyric mood*)

Yes. . . .

CLEO

Not many people are as happy as I am, not many!

STARK

Your friend, Willy Wax, is back from the coast. I saw it in the papers—

CLEO

Willy Wax, the dance director?

STARK

He's back from the coast.

CLEO

I saw his name in the files—

STARK

I do most of his work.

CLEO

What kind of teeth does he have?

STARK

(*Laughing*)

Teeth? Ordinary teeth.

CLEO

I mean he must be a nice man. He must have a beautiful mind to put on all those artistic ballet numbers. I saw that Sea Grotto number in his last picture. And then to travel by air, back and forth, here a show, there a film. . . . He must be a wonderful man, Mr. Wax!

STARK

Well, he's your friend—you ought to know.

CLEO

(*Surprised*)

Mine? I don't know Mr. Wax.

STARK

You said you knew him.

CLEO

I said so?

STARK

The first day? You said you'd come into the building to see him?

CLEO

You must be mistaken, Doctor.

STARK

(*Slowly, looking at her keenly*)

Yes . . . I must be.

CLEO

I'd never go out with a man the first time I met him. Not even Mr. Wax, as much as I admire that type of man.

STARK

Why not?

CLEO

They lose their respect for you. Didn't you know that?

STARK

No.

CLEO

You have to be very careful with most men. Not you—you're different.

STARK

Am I?

CLEO

Supremely! Men must drink too much nowadays, the things they do and say. I used to laugh when my mother told me.

STARK

What kind of woman is your mother?

CLEO

Mother . . . ? Opera singer. Was, used to be . . .

STARK

(*Measuring her*)

That's interesting. Where?

CLEO

(*Flustered*)

Where? In Europe. . . . (*Uneasily*) Didn't I ever tell you that before?

STARK

No.

CLEO

I come from a very interesting family. Don't you believe me?

STARK

I believe everything you want me to believe, Cleo . . . Cleo . . .

CLEO

Yes?

STARK

(*Slowly*)

That's a curious name . . . for a curious girl.

CLEO

May I ask you something?

STARK

Please.

CLEO

Why do you stare at me? Really, Doctor, all during the past weeks you kept looking at me as if I belong in a museum.

STARK

(*In a low voice*)

Perhaps . . . it's admiration.

102

CLEO

You're just saying that to make me feel good.

STARK

No. . . .

CLEO

You mean it?

STARK

Yes.

CLEO

Why?

STARK

(*Lamely*)

You've become very efficient. . . . Do you like it here?

CLEO

Very much. . . .

STARK

(*After a pause*)

You must excuse me if I annoyed you . . . by looking at you.

CLEO

Oh, I know it don't mean anything. Does it, Doctor?

STARK

No.

CLEO

I think you need me here. That's why I enjoy it so much. That's why I stay here. Don't you need me here?

STARK

Yes.

CLEO

Then I'll keep on staying here, Doctor, and you'll have to put me on a pension.

STARK

I'm older—I'll go first.

CLEO

There's not so much difference in our age, is there?

STARK

Some. . . .

CLEO

What does it matter? (*After a pause*) Dr. Stark, do you like me?

STARK

(*Dropping her hand*)

What?

CLEO

Do you?

STARK

Like you? (*The telephone in the office rings and startles them.* CLEO *answers it.*)

CLEO

(*On the telephone*)

Dr. Stark's office. . . . One moment please. (*To* STARK) Mrs. Stark. (CLEO *proffers the telephone to* STARK *who takes it without looking at her.*)

STARK

Hello, dear. . . . No, he hasn't come in yet—he's due any minute. . . . We can think about that later, dear. . . . I can't charge him—he's your father. . . . Yes. . . . Yes. . . . Yes, dear. . . . About ten—I won't finish with Mrs. Harris till after eight. . . . Yes. . . . Good-bye, dear. (STARK *returns to the waiting room, looking at his pocket watch*) I forgot about it: my father-in-law's a half hour late for his appointment. (CLEO *has just been hastily adjusting her undergarments.*)

CLEO

(*Wiggling a shoulder*)

I never adjust my shoulder straps or girdle in public, as some women do. God knows, it's so warm I'm practically naked underneath.

STARK

(*With surprising asperity*)

You mustn't say things like that!

CLEO

(*With quick genuine humility*)

I'm sorry if I offended. . . .

STARK

(*Immediately softer*)

For your own good, Cleo, I mean. Naïveness goes just so far.

CLEO

(*Sulkily*)

I'm not naïve.

STARK

(*After an uncomfortable pause*)

May I tell you something?

CLEO

You have a right to tell me anything. I work here; you pay—

STARK

That would be terrible, if you really thought that—

CLEO

(*Aloof*)

Tell me whatever you want. I don't care.

STARK

Not if you feel— (STARK *quickly breaks off.*
MR. PRINCE *has walked into the waiting room.*
CLEO *does not change her tired sulky attitude.*)

PRINCE

My children, good afternoon. (*Getting no response*) How am I feeling? Very secondary today.

CLEO

So am I. . . .

PRINCE

(*Sitting*)

I'm piling up a fortune. Why? To be the richest man in the cemetery! Who's coming to a stadium concert with me tonight? What nice little girl?

CLEO

Don't look at me.

STARK

You're late, Poppa. . . .

PRINCE

(*Smiling*)

By whose clock?

STARK

What's the joke?

PRINCE

You can't be in your right brains if you think someone can come early in such weather. Nicht wahr?

STARK

I can't give you another appointment today.

PRINCE

So another day! (*Turning to* CLEO) How is Miss Cleo? Grumpy?

CLEO

(*Shortly*)

No.

PRINCE

A teenchy-weenchy bit? (*After a pause*) I'm talking in a sea shell. Nobody answers. All because I came ten minutes late.

STARK

(*Very annoyed*)

Forty. I can't do anything in twenty—

PRINCE

I told you—another day. And how is your little affair going, between you two? (STARK *stares at* PRINCE *and turns away.*)

CLEO

It's too hot for such things.

108

PRINCE

That's right. If it was colder you'd be right in his arms. That's the beauty of cold weather: comfort.

CLEO

Nobody ever knows what you're talking about, Mr. Prince. (*Answering a look from* STARK) Well, they don't! Do you?

PRINCE

I invite you to come and listen to Jascha Heifetz tonight. Don't you understand that?

STARK

She's right . . . nobody ever knows when you're serious.

PRINCE

(*To* STARK)

You go take a walk around the block and she'll soon find out how serious I am. (*Then he laughs his remark away.*)

STARK

(*To* CLEO)

Put Mr. Prince down for another appointment, tomorrow, the same time. (CLEO *goes into the office to do so.*)

PRINCE

Did Belle put bugs into your ear?

STARK

About what?

PRINCE

I thought maybe she wanted payment in advance, to put in two gold inlays.

STARK

Belle didn't say a word.

PRINCE

(*Looking down at a newspaper*)
They expect trouble—they'll get it.

CLEO

(*Entering*)

Who?

PRINCE

Those Japs. (*Looking up at* STARK *keenly*) Belle didn't tell you not to work on my teeth without pay?

STARK

(*Irritably*)

Belle has other things to think about, Poppa!

PRINCE

(*Turning to* CLEO)

Learn an object lesson from life. You want to irritate a man?—Tell him the truth. Remember this for the time you get married.

CLEO

I don't intend to get married. It's too sordid.

PRINCE

Not with an older man. (*Winking*) Why don't you marry me, Miss Cleo? (*To* STARK *who goes to the office door*) Where are you going, Benny? Humilified by my remarks?

STARK

(*Taking the lavatory key from a hook*)

No. (STARK *gives him a look of irritation and exits, left.*)

PRINCE

Hmm . . . humilified.

CLEO

No wonder. You say such foolish things to him.

PRINCE

(*Glancing out at the Hotel Algiers*)

You like him?

CLEO

(*Defiantly*)

He's a very nice man.

PRINCE

But he lost his enterprise, years ago. He's no more resourceful. I offered to put him in a swell office—he could become a big specialist—but he likes it here.

CLEO

Why?

PRINCE

Afraid, no courage. My good daughter made him like that—afraid to take a chance. Keep what you got—"A half a loaf is better . . ." In life, my child, you must go forward. And if you don't go forward, where are you? Backward!

CLEO

You're trying to impress me. But I think you should help everybody you can. You don't have long to live—you're an old man.

PRINCE

(*With a grand flourish*)

Miss Cleo, you're talking to a man with a body like silk. Every year he takes the waters at Saratoga. He possesses the original teeth, every one! (*As* CLEO *laughs*) In all the multitudes of your acquaintanceship you won't find a man with younger ideas than your present speaker. How old are you, my child?

CLEO

How old do I look?

PRINCE

(*Ignoring her interpolation*)

I am speaking to you from wisdom, with a voice of velvet, as a past master of a Masonic Lodge: consort with an older man. In short, use your brains!

CLEO

It's lucky for me I don't take you serious. You're the biggest kidder on earth.

PRINCE

(*Smiling*)

Don't my young ideas reach out to your young ideas?

CLEO

(*Emphatically*)

I think you're flirting with me, that's all.

PRINCE

(*Winking*)

You see, you understand me to perfection! Tonight Heifetz is playing a piece by a famous author—

CLEO

I don't care for that.

PRINCE

Tomorrow night . . .

CLEO

Where?

PRINCE

You say where.

CLEO

Do you like me?

PRINCE

Truth is stranger than fiction: yes!

CLEO

(*Studying him*)

Where would you take me?

PRINCE

Anywhere. You're a girl like candy, a honey-dew melon—a delicious girl. Yes, I like you. (*After a pause, the veins suddenly standing out on his face*) I'm serious . . . do you understand that? I'm very serious, Miss Cleo. I'm talking to you from the roots up!

CLEO

(*Hesitantly*)

I'd have to tell Dr. Stark.

PRINCE

What would I have against that? Yes, you give me pleasure, Miss Cleo—just to talk.

114

CLEO

I'm glad you appreciate talk.

PRINCE

Why?

CLEO

Because you won't get more, Mr. Prince.

PRINCE

My child, it suits me to a T. (STARK *enters, his manner restrained, hangs up the key.*)

PRINCE

Look at her, Benny! Isn't she beautiful? Womanhood is fermenting through her veins. Am I wrong? (*Getting a blank look from* STARK) Don't look so humilified.

CLEO

(*With sudden discovery*)

Why do you wear high heels?!

PRINCE

I don't like to be so small. Now I go, I go, but to return. Until tomorrow . . . to both of you. Good-bye.

CLEO

Good-bye, Mr. Prince. (PRINCE *exits. Silence.*)

STARK

What did he mean by that?

CLEO

(*Defiantly*)

He dated me up—we're going out tomorrow night.

STARK

(*Coldly*)

That doesn't seem very wise to me.

CLEO

(*As coldly*)

It's my personal life.

STARK

(*Not knowing what else to say*)

Did you call the lab about the porcelain jackets for Mrs. Harris?

CLEO

(*Righteously*)

They're on the way over, Dr. Stark.

STARK

(*Starting for the office*)

I suppose you know what you're doing.

CLEO

You can be sure that I do.

STARK

Perhaps you'd better go out and eat an early supper before Mrs. Harris gets here.

CLEO

I'm not hungry.

STARK

Why are you so perverse? Otherwise you'll have to wait—

CLEO

Who's perverse, Dr. Stark?

STARK

Sometimes you irritate me.

CLEO

I suppose I have to listen to you—

STARK

No, go out and eat.

CLEO

I won't. You're blaming me for something I didn't do.

STARK

Blaming you?

CLEO

Aren't you? You have thoughts in your head and then you blame me because you have them.

STARK

What thoughts?

CLEO

(*In a defiant outburst*)

You're jealous! (*This statement momentarily paralyzes* STARK. *In that moment* FRENCHY *abruptly pokes his head in at the door, left.*)

FRENCHY

Pisst! I got a customer. (*He ducks out again.* STARK *goes to the door, quickly closes it and turns back to* CLEO, *lowering his voice.*)

STARK

(*Angrily*)

I'm . . . you're making it very difficult for me, Cleo. I'm trying to keep you on here. You're not the most efficient girl in the world—

CLEO

(*Breaking in*)

I'll leave any time you say!

STARK

I didn't say that—

CLEO

(*At bay*)

I don't have to work. My family has more money than we know what to do with. One of my brothers is at West Point—

STARK

And I suppose your father's a senator!

CLEO

What?

STARK

Why do you lie! After all, we're not all nitwits around here!

CLEO

What? . . . (STARK *falls off into angry silence, wagging his head. And* CLEO *is stopped, completely. Silence.*)

STARK

(*Finally seeing her flushed desperate face*)

I'm sorry I said that.

CLEO

(*Desperately*)

You don't believe me!

STARK

(*Gruffly, but apologetically, going to her*)

Yes, I do. Listen, Cleo, you're an unhappy lonely girl—

CLEO

(*Moving away*)

No!

STARK

But after all—

CLEO

No, you don't! Keep your hands off!

STARK

(*Genuinely contrite*)

I'm sorry if I hurt your feelings.

CLEO

I'll change my clothes and get right out!

STARK

No, you mustn't—

CLEO

Please stand out of my way.

STARK

Just a minute—

CLEO

I can't listen to you.

STARK

(*Holding her and shaking her despite himself*)
You know you tell stories, Cleo.

CLEO

(*Trying to loosen herself*)
You're stronger than I am.

STARK

Calm down a moment.

CLEO

I won't! Let me go! Please—you'd better do
it—! (STARK *suddenly releases her. She starts away
from him but stumbles and falls. She begins to get
up but starts to cry instead, remaining on the
floor.*)

STARK

(*Melted*)
Oh, my dear girl . . . !

CLEO

No! (*Weeping*) Keep away. . . . (CLEO *weeps
bitterly.* STARK *stands off balance, not knowing
what to do. He walks to the outer door, stands
there, comes back.* CLEO *slowly gets up and sits on
a chair.*)

CLEO

(*Finally, quietly*)

I'll change my uniform and go.

STARK

You know you need the job. . . .

CLEO

(*Tearfully*)

You never show anyone they're wrong by show-ing them you're right. Don't you know that? Don't you? Does it make you a great man to tell me I'm a liar? I know I'm a liar!

STARK

(*Gently, going to her*)

Cleo, I'm your friend . . . please believe me. (*She permits him to take one of her hands*) Every-one tells little fables, Cleo. Sometimes to them-selves, sometimes to others. Life is so full of brutal facts . . . we all try to soften them by making believe.

CLEO

(*Tearfully*)

You're talking of somebody else.

STARK

We all like to have good opinions of ourselves. That's why we squirm around and tell stories and adjust ourselves. It's a way to go on living proudly—

CLEO

I don't care to talk about it!

STARK

Why, I lie, myself, a dozen times a day. You can tell me anything, Cleo. (*After a silent pause*) Where do you come from?

CLEO

(*Defiantly*)

Madison Avenue! No more! I don't care to think. Sometimes I wish I didn't have a head. Last night I didn't have a wink of sleep. (*With sudden vehemence*) Nobody loves me! Millions of people moving around the city and nobody cares if you live or die. Go up a high building and see them down below. Some day I'll fall down on them all!

STARK

(*Gently*)

Is that a right thing to say?

CLEO

My home life is fearful—eight in one apartment. My father had a very hard life; he ran the store. He, my father, he shrinked—shrank?—what is it?

STARK

(*Not sure*)

Shrunk or shrank.

CLEO

My father got littler and littler . . . and one morning he died right in bed while everyone was sleeping. Mom and Gert and two married sisters and their husbands and babies—eight in one apartment! I tell them I want to be a dancer—everybody laughs. I make believe they're not my sisters. They don't know anything—they're washed out, bleached . . . everybody forgets how to dream. . . .

STARK

I understand. . . .

CLEO

That's the biggest joke around the house: "Cleo, the dancer—the Queen of Sheba!" My sister Gert's a garment worker. We share one room. She's keeping company—she comes in late. I never sleep. I have all the inconvenience of love with none of the pleasure.

STARK

Yes. . . . You're tired. Go home. I won't need you tonight.

CLEO

(*Wanly*)

I never go home if there's another place—here, the office, I mean. Where can you go? Sit in the park till it's time to go to bed?

STARK

The park is nice, cool—

CLEO

Don't you know they molest you there? You're naïve. Even policemen. (*With sudden fresh strength*) Would you laugh if I told you I want to be a dancer? Would you? Or an actress?

STARK

I certainly wouldn't!

CLEO

I like you very much!

STARK

Do you?

CLEO

Now don't smile!

STARK

(*Earnestly*)

I'm not.

CLEO

You're kind and you're good. But you're not resourceful or enterprising . . . don't smile.

STARK

No. . . .

CLEO

You're too used to this life—you lost your ambition. (*Insistently*) I must ask you not to smile and seem foolish! (*After waiting*) You don't go *out* to things any more. You move away instead of going to it. It's your wife's fault.

STARK

Is it?

CLEO

Don't you see it is? You're evasive and sideways. Where's your courage, Dr. Stark?

STARK

Courage for what?

CLEO

To go out to things, to new experiences. (*Rapidly*) My mother's always trying to hold me back, not to have all the experiences I can. Those people think you can live on good advice. Don't you think life is to live all you can and experience everything? Isn't that the only way you can develop to

126

be a real human being? Shouldn't a wife help a man do that? (*Excited by her own flow*) They won't hold me back. Their idea is to get married and have babies right away. I want babies, three or four—!

STARK

Do you?

CLEO

Sure. I'm healthy enough to have a dozen!

STARK

Are you?

CLEO

Sure, but there's time for them. Must they come the first year? Is that refined? (*Pausing to catch her breath*) Well, as I was saying, no good comes out of good advice, even if it's good. And that's how your wife broke up your courage—

STARK

(*Breaking in*)

Don't you think you're going too far?

CLEO

(*Not to be stopped now*)

If you expect to find out about me, you must expect me to find out about you.

STARK

Okay, but don't you think you have arbitrary opinions?

CLEO

(*Emphatically*)

No! (*Then*) What does that mean, arbitrary?

STARK

You're hungry for expression, Cleo. That makes you talk sometimes without thinking too much about what you're saying. But don't ever hesitate to say what's on your mind. . . . I like to hear it.

CLEO

Yes? . . . Well, I don't like your wife.

STARK

Why?

CLEO

(*After a pause, shyly*)

I love you!

STARK

(*After a pause, in a low voice*)

You're a fanciful girl. . . .

CLEO

Did you hear what I said?

128

STARK

No. . . .

CLEO

(*In a low voice*)

Do you want me to say it again?

STARK

No.

CLEO

And now you smile again. . . . (*They suddenly stop their conversation.* COOPER *has entered the waiting room, seeing nothing, his mind completely on his own troubles and the heat. He is too hot and discomfited to sit, prowling around instead.*)

COOPER

They're frying eggs on the sidewalk. The public is staggering around. (*At the water cooler*) Municipal champagne . . . ah-cha-cha!

CLEO

(*Making conversation*)

People in the city have a sweet kind of dizziness in the summer time, don't they?

COOPER

Maybe you, Cleo, not me. (*Flopping down heavily*) God was smart. He promised no more floods—

129

He knew fire was a worse way. (*Getting up and prowling to the window, right*) How are your petunias doing here?

STARK

(*Over-casual*)

I forgot to water them today.

CLEO

(*Quickly, with veiled pride*)

I did it before, Dr. Stark. . . .

STARK

(*As above*)

Did you? Thank you, Cleo.

CLEO

(*With a glance in* COOPER's *direction*)

You're welcome, Dr. Stark.

STARK

(*As above*)

They don't seem to do so well there.

CLEO

They look just like orphan babies. I feel so sorry for them.

COOPER

(Mopping his brow)

Fire, fire—fire in the church. (*He sits again and picks up a newspaper. Indicating the newspaper*) According to this man, the katydids began to sing this week, across the Hudson. (*Bitterly*) Everybody should rejoice . . . it means an early frost, he says.

CLEO

With all this heat, I don't see how anyone could have the nerve to predict that.

COOPER

(Heavily, throwing the paper aside)

What does it cost him to predict . . .

STARK

(Sympathetically)

Rest, Phil, take it easy.

COOPER

(Snorting)

Rest! Who rests in the front-line trench? I suddenly realized life is a war . . . for forty years it never entered my mind.

CLEO

What kind of war?

COOPER

You expect me to explain forty-one years in a minute?

CLEO

(*Naïvely*)

Take more than a minute. . . .

COOPER

Cleo, take a number from one to ten. You got it? Add three, divide by four. You got it . . . throw it away! Ah—cha-cha! (*There is a pause of silence which comes from both* STARK *and* CLEO *being frightened and discomfited by* COOPER'S *mood. Finally* COOPER *stops fanning himself with the newspaper and starts across to the water cooler for another drink.* STARK *catches* CLEO *looking at him earnestly.* CLEO *covers up by shifting her glance to the water cooler.*)

CLEO

It's nice how a cooler keeps giving water. You press a button—

COOPER

If only they invented hydrants in the streets which give out milk and honey! . . . we'd be happier people. (*Turning to them with new belligerence*) Don't I try? Can anyone accuse me of indifference to my work? Why can't I make a living? I'm falling apart by inches. (*Suddenly sobbing*) Where can I sail away? To where? I'm ashamed to live! An ostrich can hide his head. Diphtheria gets more respect than me! They coddle germs in laboratories—they feed the white mice twice a day. . . . Why don't somebody coddle *me*? (*Controlling himself now*) What did I do to my fellow man? Why am I punished like this? (*Trembling again on the brink of sobs, but holding them back*) Where is the God they told me about? Why should an innocent boy and an old lady suffer? I ask you to tell me, what is the Congress doing? Where are they in the hour of the needs of the people? (*Appealing to* STARK *personally*) Did you ever see such times? Where will it end if they can't use millions of Coopers? Why can't they fit me in, a man of my talents? The sick ones walk the streets, the doctors sit at home. Where, where is it? What is it? . . . what, what, what? . . . (COOPER *trickles off into silence.* CLEO *and* STARK *can be only helplessly silent in the face of this emotional speech. After* COOPER *blows his nose and wipes his eyes, a little ashamed of his feeling, he says with a faint bitter smile, mocking himself*) Gaze on the Columbia University lunatic! The warrior of Ypres and Verdun! . . . (*He moves his trembling hand across his brow, at the same time taking a card from his pocket and handing it to* STARK.)

STARK

(*Of the card*)

What is this, Phil?

COOPER

I came just now from being registered. I'm classified—you're talking to type four.

STARK

(*Puzzled, turning the card over*)

I don't see what—

COOPER

Blood.

CLEO

(*Moving forward*)

What?

COOPER

(*With self-mockery*)

I decided to become a blood donor on the side.

CLEO

(*Horrified*)

Oh, no!

COOPER

They pay well, thirty dollars a pint.

134

CLEO

(*In a low voice*)

A pint's a lot of blood, Dr. Cooper. . . .

COOPER

A boy there gave fifteen times last year: a young fortune. He told me he lives on a plain diet, onions and bread, no meats or anything.

STARK

(*After a pause*)

Phil . . . you mean it?

COOPER

(*Bitterly*)

They didn't want me at first. But it seems I'm a type everybody needs . . . I'm a very common type.

STARK

Phil, you don't mean that!

COOPER

Why not? It's a legitimate business, like pressing pants or cleaning fish.

CLEO

(*Trying to be helpful*)

I think he's joking, Dr. Stark. (*Now* COOPER *turns and unleashes the wrath of many weeks on* CLEO's *head.*)

COOPER

Why don't you mind your business! Who do you think you are? Keep your mouth shut around here, Miss Smarty! Learn to mind your lousy business! (COOPER *abruptly starts right, as if to his office.* CLEO *and* STARK *sit, frozen. Just as abruptly* COOPER *now returns. He walks right up to* CLEO, *tears in eyes, wrathfully shaking his fist in her face again. She stands motionless, pale, tragic.* STARK *scrambles to his feet, about to get between the other two. But now* COOPER *suddenly drops his fist and throws his arms around* CLEO. *She, crying, does likewise.* COOPER *kisses her and breaks away.*)

CLEO

(*Crying*)

Stay here, Dr. Cooper. Sit down. Don't go out, Doct— (*But* COOPER *is gone, plunged off through the door, left. There is a further silence.* STARK *has no words.* CLEO *slowly sits, crying a little.* STARK *crosses and sits by her side, stroking her hair.*)

STARK

(*Softly*)

Don't cry, dear. . . .

CLEO

(*Shaking her head*)

No. . . . (*Now no longer crying, head up*) I feel so sorry for Dr. Cooper. . . .

STARK

You mustn't mind what he said.

CLEO

He'll hurt himself.

STARK

A man with that sense of responsibility for his family? No. . . .

CLEO

Are you sure?

STARK

Yes. . . .

CLEO

I understand his feelings. . . . He's all alone in the world. Nobody wants him . . . like an orphan.

STARK

I wish I could give you an idea of his talent.

CLEO

Better than you?

STARK

He always was.

CLEO

(*Quickly*)

Don't say that. (*She draws her hand away from his.*)

137

STARK

Well, some people don't agree with me.

CLEO

Who don't?

STARK

You don't. My wife, she—

CLEO

(*Starting up, fresh and indestructible*)

Don't mention her to me! And let Dr. Cooper be better than you, but don't tell me. I never want to hear those things.

STARK

(*Slowly standing*)

Why? . . .

CLEO

You're asking me why again? I told you why before. . . . (*They look at each other in silence. Finally:*)

STARK

We both must forget what was said before. . . .

CLEO

(*Coolly, intently*)

You don't love your wife. . . .

138

STARK

You mustn't say that!

CLEO

(*As above*)

If you did . . . would you let me talk this way?

STARK

(*Flustered*)

Forget it, Cleo!

CLEO

(*Defiantly*)

I won't forget it.

STARK

(*Hardly audible*)

This is an office. I'm a married man. . . . You know I'm a married man, don't you?

CLEO

Just because you're sad you can't make me sad. No one can. I have too much in me!

STARK

You're wonderful. . . .

CLEO

(*Almost dancing*)

Talent!—I'm talented. I don't know for what, but it makes me want to dance in my bones! Don't want to be lonely, never left alone! Why should I cry? I have a throat to sing with, a heart to love with! Why don't you love me, Dr. Stark? I was ten, then fifteen— I'm almost twenty now. Everything is in a hurry and you ought to love me.

STARK

Cleo, please. . . .

CLEO

You're good, you're kind, you're like a father. Do you love your wife? I'm intuitive— I know you don't!

STARK

(*Making a last effort to stop her*)

Cleo!

CLEO

We're *both* alone, so alone. You might be like Cooper in a year or two. Maybe I lie. You know why. Because I'm alone—nobody loves me. But I won't have it that way. I'll change life.

STARK

You're wonderful. . . .

CLEO

You don't deserve me. Not you or any other man I ever met.

STARK

(*In an agony of indecision*)

Cleo, dear. . . .

CLEO

(*Shyly*)

I'll call you Benny in a minute! (*After a throb of hesitation*) Ben! Benny! . . . (*They are standing off from each other, poised on needles*) Don't be afraid. . . .

STARK

. . . No? . . .

CLEO

Love me. . . . Love me, Ben.

STARK

. . . Can't do that. . . .

CLEO

(*Moving forward a step*)

Put your arms up and around me.

STARK

Cleo. . . . (*Now they move in on each other. Everything else gone, they are together in a full, fierce embrace, together in a swelter of heat, mis-understanding, loneliness and simple sex.)*

Curtain

ACT TWO

SCENE II

PLACE: *The same.*
TIME: *The beginning of August.*

The waiting room is empty. The electric fan buzzes monotonously, matching the sound of the dentist's drill within STARK'S *operating room. Through his glass door we see moving shadows. A newspaper rattles on the chair every time the fan moves that way. It is late afternoon; soon the brazen day will cool off into quiet evening.*

The telephone rings. CLEO *comes out of the operating room to answer it. She is hurriedly and tensely followed by* STARK. *He speaks in a low voice, not wanting to be heard by his patient.*

STARK

If that's my wife, I'll speak to her.

CLEO

(*Stopping and shrugging her shoulders*)
Speak to her . . . what do I care?

STARK

(*In a low voice*)
Cleo. . . . (*She turns away from him. The telephone rings again.* STARK *hastens to it*) Hello? . . . Oh, yes . . . yes. . . . (*Returning to* CLEO) My father-in-law. For you.

CLEO

For me?

STARK

He wants to speak to you.

CLEO

(*Staring at him*)
To me?

STARK

Yes. (*They look at each other a moment, she crossly. Then she starts for the telephone, but he stops her timidly, awkwardly, almost nervously.*)

STARK

Don't be angry, Cleo.

143

CLEO
(Impatiently)

I'm not.

STARK

Yesterday, when she called, you told her I was busy. It's all I heard from her last night.

CLEO

Oh, your wife.

PATIENT
(From within)

Can I smoke a cigar?

STARK
(Calling out to the patient)

Just let that dry a minute, Mr. Wax. (*To* CLEO) After all, we don't want her to—

CLEO
(In a final burst)

You must think that's all I have to do, think about your wife. (CLEO *pulls away from him, going to the telephone. For a moment* STARK *watches her and then returns to his patient, closing the door behind him.*)

CLEO

(*On the telephone*)

This is Cleo. (*After a pause*) That's very nice, but I can't go. (*Listens*) Because. . . . Because why? I don't like that kind of music. . . . I don't care if it's the best seats, Mr. Prince. (*Listens*) No. . . . Maybe some other time. . . . I think once a week is enough to go out with an old man. Anyway, I have a date. (*Listens*) Yes, next week . . . yes. 'Bye. (CLEO *indolently comes out into the waiting room. She has been making a display of temper with* STARK, *but she is really enjoying her life in the office.* PRINCE *is pursuing her,* WILLY WAX *is inside—she is busy and excited. Now she adjusts her damp underclothing. She catches sight of herself in the wall mirror to which she draws closer. She waves her hands, poises herself in a dancing position, shakes out her hair. Suddenly she turns with a start.* FRENCHY *has been standing at the door for a few seconds*) You frightened me!

FRENCHY

I'm a boogey man. (*He drinks from the cooler*) You were getting quite enthusiastic about yourself, there in the mirror.

CLEO

(*Sarcastically*)

I like myself, Dr. Jensen.

FRENCHY

So it seems, Goldilocks.

CLEO

Anyone can see I'm not a blonde.

FRENCHY

(*Looking her over frankly*)

All the girls are Goldilocks to me. Is the Doc busy?

CLEO

Yes.

FRENCHY

Any picture magazines in there? (*Without waiting for an answer* FRENCHY *goes into the office, where he rummages around.* CLEO *goes to the water cooler for a drink.* STARK *opens his door and looks out. Seeing she is alone he crosses the waiting room and speaks to her in a low voice.*)

STARK

Cleo. . . . Wax is leaving the chair. Don't go out with him. . . .

CLEO

I'd better wait till I'm asked.

STARK

Don't, for my sake. . . . (FRENCHY *is standing in the office doorway, taking in this little pri-*

vate drama. CLEO *signals to* STARK *that* FRENCHY
is there. STARK *turns and sees they are not alone.*)

STARK

(*Hurriedly*)

Oh, you, Frenchy. Be with you in five minutes.
(FRENCHY *waves to the retreating* STARK, *who
exits, closing the operating-room door behind him.*
FRENCHY *comes down into the waiting room,
perusing the magazine in his hands.*)

FRENCHY

(*Softly*)

You oughta be careful . . . there's a soft shoulder ahead.

CLEO

I don't know what that means.

FRENCHY

(*With a smoothing-out gesture*)

You might go off the road— (*Without another
word* CLEO *starts for the operating room.*)

FRENCHY

(*Blocking her way*)

Wait a minute, don't give me that flight-of-the-
bumble-bee stuff!

147

CLEO

(*Haughtily*)

I beg your pardon?

FRENCHY

Who's in there?

CLEO

(*Coldly*)

A very distinguished gentleman . . . which you are not.

FRENCHY

Who?

CLEO

Mr. Wax, Mr. Willy Wax, the dance director.

FRENCHY

He ain't even distinguished to his mother!

CLEO

(*Loftily*)

A man who gets his name in the paper so often must be important to some people.

FRENCHY

(*Warningly*)

You got a lot to learn, Cleo. What's between you?

148

CLEO

"Between you?" Who?

FRENCHY

Or don't you speak without your lawyer? (*Coming up closer to her and dropping his voice*) Listen, don't twist Stark's head. He's foolish, but he's good and we like him. Don't get him in trouble. (*Taking her arm*) Come on over to my office.

CLEO

(*Pulling away*)

I'll do nothing of the sort.

FRENCHY

(*After a silent penetrating look*)

Are you honest?

CLEO

What?

FRENCHY

Do you like him?

CLEO

(*Indignantly*)

Who do you think you are? A government agent?

FRENCHY

Weave, weave patiently, thou gentle spider . . . one of these days you might get hurt.

CLEO

I would like to see you touch me. I would just like to see it!

FRENCHY

Don't forget, I see what you're up to.

CLEO

You don't see anything!

FRENCHY

Quoth the raven! Look, Cleo, for him there is sleep and day and work again. He's not a happy man. He spends his days trying to exhaust himself so he can fall asleep quick. Not that he told me this. . . . I seen it with my two good eyes. Don't make trouble for him, Cleo. Don't take him over the coals. Unless you're serious, unless you love him. . . .

CLEO

And if I do?

FRENCHY

(*Appraisingly*)

Do you? See if you can understand this: through unhappy marriage he's lost power for accomplishment—he don't get much personal satisfaction out of his work; and the man who don't get that is a lost man. Lots of things he longs for he'll never take. And like millions of others he constantly feels worried, depressed and inadequate. But!—His unhappiness is a dangerous habit of which he is not fully aware—it may make him bust loose in some curious way . . . can you be it?

CLEO

You must have read all that in a book.

FRENCHY

(*Disgusted*)

What goes on in the head of a moth?—Nothing! (*He reaches out and smacks an imaginary moth between his palms. Emphatically*) That was you, in effigy and promise!

CLEO

(*Her mood abruptly changing*)

Why don't you like me? Did I ever harm you or anyone else?

FRENCHY

Cleo, I work like an antitoxin—*before* the complications come. And I know the difference between love and pound cake. . . . (*The operating room door opens and out comes* WILLY WAX, *followed by* STARK. WAX *is a small dark man with shrewd roving eyes and a glib tongue, plus a definite tired sense of his own importance. Success has given him an unpleasant easiness. Now he is shuffling a thin panatela in his soft hands.*)

WAX

(*Twisting his face*)

Can I smoke with this materia medica in my mouth?

STARK

(*Smiling uneasily*)

Better wait ten minutes, Mr. Wax.

(*Note: One attractive woman is an entire grandstand for* WAX. *Now he plays charmingly, eruditely for* CLEO. *As for* CLEO, WAX *present, even her breasts stand at attention. Alas, she is not yet wise in the ways of the world and the creatures therein.*)

WAX

(*Affably, of* FRENCHY)

Who's this? Haven't I met you somewhere? Don't you work in the cafeteria downstairs? I'm Willy Wax.

FRENCHY

I'm Dr. Jensen.

WAX

(*Knowing who he was all the time*)

Certainly! To be sure! You did that excellent foot work for me last year. (*Appealingly*) No?

FRENCHY

(*Smiling faintly*)

Now you placed me. . . .

WAX

(*Shuffling his cigar*)

Well, I suppose I'll have to chew this cigar. I'd like to look at the x-rays, too.

STARK

(*Promptly*)

Miss Singer, please show Mr. Wax the x-rays.

CLEO

(*All attention*)

This way please, Mr. Wax.

WAX

Peculiar how I never remember names, but *never!* That comes from living alone. I have to admit I'm a lone wolf—

FRENCHY

(*Involuntarily*)

Bow wow! (WAX *gives* FRENCHY *a quick stabbing look and then follows* CLEO *into the office.* FRENCHY *smiles faintly.* STARK'S *worried eye goes after* CLEO.)

FRENCHY

(*Sotto voce*)

That boy, he'd better be a genius!

153

STARK

I'll look at that tooth now, Frenchy. (FRENCHY *and* STARK *exit to the operating room, closing the door.* WAX *comes to the office door, holding up a small strip of x-ray film, but first making sure the others are gone. Now he is alone with his prey, but gently, gently, winningly.*)

WAX

(*The tired, appealing boy*)
One needs a code for these things. No?

CLEO

(*Made nervous by his proximity*)
You see, if you hold it this way—

WAX

(*Abruptly hands them back*)
No, put them back. I'll live without them. (*Coming into the waiting room*) I'd like to smoke and I can't smoke.

CLEO

(*Sympathetically, following him out*)
It'll go away, Mr. Wax.

WAX

I'm nervous.

CLEO

Why?

154

WAX

Overworked, but definitely! Talent's a responsibility—

CLEO

Is it?

WAX

You have to work hard . . . and lead a lonely life. What's your name? First name, I mean.

CLEO

(*Shyly*)

Cleo Singer.

WAX

You're a strange girl to find in this office. No?

CLEO

Why? I'm a very efficient dental assistant—

WAX

I mean that sort of mazda glow in your eyes. (*Suddenly*) There's a fever in you! You're talented! For what?

CLEO

I don't want to spend the rest of my life in an office.

WAX

I've seen you somewhere.

CLEO

I don't think so, Mr. Wax.

WAX

(*Winningly*)
Don't be shy with me, Cleo.

CLEO

I'm not, but you have so much on your mind.
The late hours and all that, putting on shows one
after another—you're different than the other
men I know—

WAX

No, my texture is just as coarse.

CLEO

I don't know *coarse* men. . . .

WAX

Most men are. You're living in the city of the
dreadful night: a man is coarse or he doesn't sur-
vive.

CLEO

Are you married, if you don't mind my asking?

WAX

(*Sadly*)

An artist hasn't time for that, dear. Not that he wouldn't want a home and children. Are you sure I haven't seen you somewhere?

CLEO

Last week, in the elevator? I was in the back when you—

WAX

Not on a choo-choo train? Never out to the coast?

CLEO

No, I wasn't. . . .

WAX

(*Groaning*)

Movies! They're what started me off on my path of painless perversion.

CLEO

(*Sadly*)

You must be a very lonely man.

WAX

I'm nourished by my sensitivity, such as is left. (*Looking at her open eyes*) Do I glisten with arrogance, Cleo?

157

CLEO

(*Stoutly*)

I think you're one of the nicest men I ever met.

WAX

(*Sotto voce*)

Your eyes are beautiful, Cleo—fresh and alive.
Where do you eat your dinner?

CLEO

When?

WAX

Tonight, for example.

CLEO

(*Dismayed*)

Oh, I have a date tonight.

WAX

I have a better idea than that.

CLEO

What?

WAX

Have you had your lunch?

CLEO

No.

WAX

Have it with me, down my office, in twenty minutes. I won't have time to go out, but they send up sandwiches and milk.

CLEO

(*Hesitantly, looking at* STARK's *door*)
Well, I don't . . .

WAX

(*Quickly*)
Have you seen the new method of charting dances on a board? You'd like to see that . . . and then we can talk. . . .

CLEO

I'll be there, Mr. Wax. Twenty minutes?

WAX

Good. I'll tell my secretary you're coming. Do you know what I see about you, Cleo? You're looking for a Columbus to discover you— It's in your eyes. (*Going to the door*) Stewed fruit, do you like that?

CLEO

Whatever you eat, Mr. Wax.

WAX

(*With great charm*)
Come down soon. . . .

159

CLEO

Yes. . . . Good-bye.

WAX

Good-bye.

CLEO
(*Suddenly*)
Can I tell you something?

WAX
(*Smiling*)
A thousand volumes full.

CLEO

Any dance routine—if I watch it once, I can do it.

WAX

So . . . you're interested in dancing!

CLEO

Yes.

WAX

Well, we'll see if you have any talent. Good-bye for now. (WAX *exits.* CLEO *stands stock still, thrilling all over. Suddenly she flings her arms out, stretching on her toes. She is embracing the world!* FRENCHY *and* STARK *come out of the operating*

room. CLEO *sits and demurely fans herself with a
magazine.*)

STARK

I can't fix it till the swelling goes down.

FRENCHY

Yeah, but when the swelling goes down it won't
hurt.

STARK

(*His eyes on* CLEO)

That's the time to fix it.

FRENCHY

(*Agreeing*)

You're the doctor. (*Turning to leave; to* CLEO)
So long, Angel Skin.

CLEO

Don't say good-bye; you'll be back in five minutes.

FRENCHY

Yeah, Cleo, you're like a magnet!

CLEO

You're wild, Dr. Jensen—just like a sea-bird.
(FRENCHY *chortles at that and exits, right.* CLEO
and STARK *are now alone for the first time in
hours. She begins to peruse the magazine, waiting
for his advances. He watches her for a moment.*)

STARK

(*Softly, despite his several anxieties*)

"How green you are and fresh in this old world." . . . Shakespeare. (*Going to her*) Are you mad, Cleo?

CLEO

(*Pertly*)

Only dogs are mad. (*He sits down beside her and suddenly kisses her shyly.*)

CLEO

(*Coquetting*)

When I was a little girl a fortune teller told me I'd meet a man like you. (*He kisses her again*) You're a regular kissing bug.

STARK

Yes, perhaps I oughtn't to do that.

CLEO

I didn't say not to.

STARK

(*Holding her hand*)

I like to hold your hand.

CLEO

Where will we go tonight?

162

STARK

After the lecture? Well . . .

CLEO

(*Archly*)

I suppose you have to go home. Mr. Prince takes me to interesting places. You're not doing me a favor when you take me out.

STARK

The favor's all on your side, Cleo.

CLEO

Palisades Park is not my idea of heaven.

STARK

I don't know any places, Cleo. I'm not the kind of man who goes out much. You can help me find places to go. We'll go to a Eugene O'Neill play in the winter—

CLEO

You're ashamed of me.

STARK

(*Surprised*)

Why do you say that?

CLEO

You take me to out-of-the-way places—a movie

on 14th Street! You don't want people to see us together; isn't that true?

STARK

It's not shame. . . .

CLEO

You're very cautious then.

STARK

Yes. . . .

CLEO

Why are you cautious? We didn't do anything. (*After waiting for an answer*) You think about your wife all the time.

STARK

I have to, Cleo.

CLEO

Why? She doesn't think about you.

STARK

That isn't true. Maybe we could go to the Planetarium tonight. You said you wanted to see it.

CLEO

Mr. Wax was very attracted to me.

164

STARK

What did he say?

CLEO

Are you jealous?

STARK

(*Smiling*)

No.

CLEO

Then why should I tell you? Do you love me?
(*Note:* CLEO, *in her contact with those she thinks
"superior people," is often afraid of repudiation
on one score or another. This is so in her relationship with* STARK. *For this reason she seldom fully
extends the power she feels over him. This gives
most of her impulses and gestures a contained
tentative quality; an impulse is seldom fully re-
leased.*)

STARK

(*Uneasily*)

Do you want to go to the Planetarium—

CLEO

Are you listening to me?

STARK

Yes. (*He tries to take her hand.*)

165

CLEO

No, I won't let you hold my hand. (*Moving across the room*) I feel discouraged. I'd like to leave this place.

STARK

Why?

CLEO

You don't need me here. I don't make much difference in your life.

STARK

It's not fair to say that. I can't do everything I'd like to do, Cleo. (*Suddenly*) But you make me very happy, very happy!

CLEO

Do I?

STARK

Gee, yes! (*He crosses to her as if to embrace her, but* CLEO *eludes him with a laugh.*)

CLEO

Here comes that kissing bug!

STARK

You make me very happy! Let me put my arms around you.

CLEO

Nope.

STARK

Please.

CLEO

You can't creep up on me like that. You never think of me.

STARK

I thought of you all last night. I was walking on the boardwalk and I thought of you. Do you know what the waves are saying?

CLEO

What?

STARK

Your name . . .

CLEO

Well, were you walking alone?

STARK

No.

CLEO

With your wife?

STARK

Yes. . . . (*There is a pause;* CLEO *walks to the water cooler.*)

CLEO

I have some bad news temporarily.

167

STARK

(*Strained*)

What?

CLEO

I'm having lunch with Mr. Wax, down his office.

STARK

When?

CLEO

Now. Do you mind?

STARK

(*In a low voice*)

No.

CLEO

Are you jealous?

STARK

Yes.

CLEO

He's a very interesting man—I want to hear what he has to say. I can learn from him. He's interested in my dancing.

STARK

(*Miserably*)

Wax makes propaganda for Willy Wax, dear. He's interested in two things—himself and girls for himself. I know him—he's been in this building for years.

CLEO

(*Touched by his misery, softly*)

You act as if I was leaving. I'm not leaving you, Ben.

STARK

(*Pleadingly*)

Don't go down there.

CLEO

(*Earnestly*)

Don't you know you're my best friend? My *only* friend?

STARK

Being a friend is one thing. . . . (*Taking her hand*) Cleo . . . we don't belong to each other. . . . I mean I don't have the right . . . this is like living in a subway and never getting off the train. . . .

CLEO

(*Softly*)

Is it fair for you to question my motives? Is it?

STARK

Cleo. . . . (*Suddenly he kisses her hand.*)

CLEO

That's right—kiss it. And kiss the fingers, every

169

one. (*He does so*) And you do that of your own
free will. (*With sudden anxiety*) Did I offend?

STARK

No, dear, no. . . .

CLEO

You have to always remember that you belong
to me! Let me pull your nose. (*She does*) Your
ears. (*She does*) No, you can't kiss me. (*She eludes
him*) For another week, no kissing. . . . Now I
have to go.

STARK

Don't go. . . .

CLEO

I have to, Ben. Don't worry. I'll be back soon.
(STARK *releases her hand. She goes to the door.*)
Don't worry, Ben. . . . (*The door is opened by*
BELLE STARK *just in time to hear the name being
uttered by* CLEO. *To* BELLE) Ooh, you frightened
me! Excuse me, I'm going to lunch. . . . (*The
two women look at each other briefly, and* CLEO
exits.)

BELLE

She uses a very heavy perfume.

STARK

(*Over-brightly*)

Belle, I'm surprised to see you in town!

BELLE

(*Quizzically*)

But pleased?

STARK

Very pleased.

BELLE

(*Sitting*)

The beach is boring.

STARK

It must be cool down there. I wish I didn't have to stick in the office—

BELLE

(*Wanly*)

I feel like a poached egg.

STARK

Why don't you stay down there, dear? It's cool, you can rest—

BELLE

(*Wearily*)

Don't be funny, Ben! A place is not a place. A place is who you're with!

STARK

(*Meekly, wondering what she knows*)

Unfortunately, I have this lecture tonight, at the Clinic. But I'll be down early in the afternoon, tomorrow . . . tomorrow? . . . Yes, Saturday, and we'll have the whole week-end together.

BELLE

A week-end starts on Friday in the summer. If you saw the other husbands at the beach today you'd know it. (*Suddenly she almost sobs, but immediately catches herself.* STARK *is immediately at her side, his arm around her shoulder. He is both touched and uneasy, a little sick at heart.*)

STARK

(*Gently*)

Is that why you came to town, dear? You felt alone?

BELLE

(*Dry-eyed*)

Yes.

STARK

Why don't you have Milly Heitner down till I get there? They can use the other room—I'll move the table out—

BELLE

Milly and Jack are in San Diego, California.

STARK

I forgot that. . . . (*After a pause*) Would you want to stay in town tonight? . . .

BELLE

Do you want me to?

STARK

I wouldn't ask if I didn't. (*Seeing her distressed face*) What's the matter, Belle?

BELLE

Your heart is so faint, the way you ask. Am I being a pest?

STARK

You're not a pest, Belle.

BELLE

For God's sake, tell me if I am. I'll go back to the beach and bury myself in the sand up to the chin!

STARK

(*Meekly*)

I was only thinking— I have that lecture to-night. . . . (*Now* BELLE *begins to flirt with her husband, an activity which does not become her. But she is desperate. The flirting comes out thin, pitiful, dry and nervous. To both of them it is an extremely painful interlude.*)

BELLE

Aren't you afraid I'll leave you, Ben? Down there at the beach, alone? All day long? Suppose an interesting man came along? Don't you care?

STARK

(*Smiling uneasily*)

You won't run away, dear. . . .

BELLE

(*Half smiling*)

I might . . . or don't you think I'm attractive enough for a man—

STARK

You're as attractive as you ever were, Belle.

BELLE

Confess to your wife—aren't you ever afraid to leave her alone as much as you do?

STARK

(*Shaking a finger at her*)

Send me a wire before you elope. (*They both laugh weakly.*)

BELLE

(*Fishing for affirmations*)

You'd *like* to get rid of me.

STARK

Never, never!

BELLE

Admit it—

174

STARK

Never, dear, not for a day. . . . And I don't want you to talk that way, even in a joke.

BELLE

(*Suddenly*)

I'll make you an offer, Ben. Why don't I take this job?

STARK

This . . .

BELLE

(*Quickly*)

I'd get my typing back in no time. In one week I'd have this office on an efficient working basis. . . .

STARK

You don't mean it.

BELLE

Yes, I do.

STARK

(*Dubiously*)

You wouldn't want this job.

BELLE

Why not? I'm loyal, honest—you'd get me cheap—

STARK

A wife in her husband's office? I need a girl here who can take orders. She has to clean instruments, be yelled at, be impersonal—

BELLE

I can be impersonal.

STARK

Why do you bring up a thing like that, after all these years?

BELLE

Why are you so outraged?

STARK

(*Angrily*)

Who's outraged?

BELLE

Isn't your tone unreasonable?

STARK

Isn't your request? In all fairness . . . Well, I see your point, Belle, but I give in to you on many things. Gee, I know it's no bed of roses for you, but a man's office is his castle—

BELLE

I can be as impersonal as some snip of a girl with vaseline on her eyelids. I want you to fire her and let me—

STARK

Yes? Well, I won't do it!

BELLE

Why does she call you Ben, that little papoose?

STARK

What?

BELLE

I heard her call you Ben when I came in. Is that a habit of hers?

STARK

I didn't notice that.

BELLE

Ask her to call you Dr. Stark—do me the favor. Or would that be straining relationships too much?

STARK

(*Quickly*)

What relationships?

BELLE

(*Acidly*)

Any which might exist. Secondly, I intend to go to that lecture tonight.

STARK

That doesn't frighten me.

BELLE

Will she be there?

STARK

She takes notes.

BELLE

Notes? Will they be printed in a book, "Confessions of a Dentist"?

STARK

Belle, I deplore these suspicions!

BELLE

Let her go or you'll confirm them!

STARK

(*Going to her after a pause*)

Belle, can you stand there and seriously tell me . . .

178

BELLE

(*Eluding him*)

Off . . . the scrawny shoulders, my dental friend. Now make up your mind, Ben. . . .

STARK

(*Blazing out*)

Will you stop that stuff for a change! It's about time you began to realize there are two ends to a rope. *I* have needs, too! This one-way street has to end! I'm not going to stay under water like an iceberg the rest of my life. You've got me licked—I must admit it. All right, I'm sleeping, I don't love you enough. But what do *you* give? What do you know about *my* needs?

BELLE

Don't you dare speak that way to me!

STARK

You've been speaking like that for ten years!

BELLE

You won't throw me away for that dirty rag of a girl!

STARK

The hell with the girl! I'm talking of us. . . .

179

BELLE

(*Wildly*)

I gave you too much of my life for that. You've used me up. . . .

STARK

Belle, for Pete's sake . . . !

BELLE

And now you want to throw me off. But you're a man, not an animal—you can't do that!

STARK

If you can't talk facts, keep quiet!

BELLE

(*Weeping*)

My mother sat crying by the window for twenty years—

STARK

Every word is nonsense!

BELLE

But you can't do that to me. I wasn't born in Europe— I'm a modern woman— I don't weep, not me. . . . (*She trails off into silence.* STARK *gruffly hands her a handkerchief, which she uses.*)

STARK

(Bitterly)

Sonofagun. . . .

BELLE

Not weep, not weep. . . . (BELLE *turns scornfully and enters the office, slamming the door in* STARK'S *following face.*)

STARK

(At the door)

No, open the door, Belle. Open it. *(Rattling and turning the knob)* Unlock the door, Belle. *(Twisting the knob again)* Belle? . . . Belle? . . . Let me in. . . . (DR. COOPER *now enters the waiting room.* STARK *quickly walks away from the door.*)

COOPER

Just the man I'm looking for.

STARK

Hello, Phil.

COOPER

I came in today for one express purpose. *(He sees* BELLE'S *shadow moving on the glass of the closed office door)* What is that shadow in there, moving?

STARK

(Gloomily)

My wife. . . .

COOPER

(*Calling jovially*)

Come out of hiding, Mrs. Stark. Phil Cooper's got a surprise. (*Draws a check from his pocket, followed by fountain pen*) See Phil Cooper create a historical moment, like the signing of the Declaration of Independence. (*Signing the check on the back*) A check for thirty dollars and I now sign it over to you. (*Calling over his shoulder*) Come out, Mrs. Stark, and see history in the making.

STARK

She has a little headache.

COOPER

What can take it away easier? (*Handing it over to* STARK) There it is. . . . A first payment, on account. (BELLE *now stands in the doorway, outwardly calm and collected*) Look what I gave your spouse, Mrs. Stark. (*Laughingly*) Blood money!

STARK

(*To* BELLE)

You can bank that, dear. (*He extends the check to her, a peace offering, but she rejects it, saying with a coolness which* COOPER *doesn't notice.*)

BELLE

Bank it yourself. (*Rebuked and hurt,* STARK *silently folds the check and puts it in his wallet.* BELLE *goes for her purse and gloves.*)

STARK

(*Sullenly*)

Where are you going?

BELLE

(*Coldly*)

Home, to my palace on the beach.

STARK

(*Trying to stop her*)

Belle, listen—

BELLE

You're such an actor, Ben. Good-bye, Dr. Cooper.

COOPER

Good-bye. (BELLE *exits, leaving* STARK *feeling foolish and angry. Joyfully*) I'm hot, but who can blame me for that? (*Drinking at the water cooler*) Nature makes the heat and the heat eats me up. What am I to Nature?—A hot dog on a roll! Say, a few more transfusions and I'll dream it's better days. (*Turning to face* STARK) Stark?

183

STARK

What? (COOPER's *answer is to look at* STARK, *then step forward and kiss him on the cheek.*)

COOPER

Imagine what a kiss you would get if I paid the *whole* debt! (*And* COOPER *has exited happily through the door, left.* STARK *stands there angrily thoughtful. He wags his head angrily, strides around the room several times. Finally he looks out of the window, examining the Hotel Algiers. A sense of resolution grows into his appearance. Suddenly he puts his hand to his heart, not having noticed before how strongly it is beating. Now* CLEO *enters, defiantly pushing open the door,* WAX *behind her.* STARK *turns on them, momentarily unnerved.*)

WAX

(*Gayly*)

Stark, what kind of hold have you got on this girl? Couldn't keep her down my office—said she had to be back—

CLEO

(*Breaking in*)

Dr. Stark has no hold on me. I have some work to do.

WAX

(*To* STARK)

I call Cleo the Radium Girl—gives off heat and light.

STARK

(*Foolishly*)

Yes. . . .

WAX

Take back the precious capsule, Stark.

CLEO

(*Annoyed*)

I wish you wouldn't say that!

WAX

Say what?

CLEO

Hinting—as if I belong to him. (WAX *looks from one to the other, understanding their relationship in a flash.*)

WAX

I beg your pardon, Cleo; that never crossed my mind.

STARK

(*Darkly*)

What never crossed your mind?

WAX

We're getting mixed up here, aren't we?

STARK

Not at all.

WAX

Come to see me again, Cleo. Or I'll call you.

CLEO

Yes.

WAX

Why are your brows bulging, Stark?

STARK

What?

WAX

(*Pleasantly*)

See you soon. (*He exits. After a momentary silence* CLEO *goes to the door, beginning to pin it back.*)

STARK

Close the door.

CLEO

(*Fretfully*)

It's hot.

STARK

I know, but close it. . . . (CLEO *closes the door, struck by* STARK's *resolute manner. Her out-*

ing to WAX'*s office has been a dismal failure. Her mind has been up here with* STARK *and* BELLE *all the time. She is nervous and defiant now, even feeling unwanted, a feeling which motivates much that she does.*)

CLEO

(*Defiantly*)

I suppose you want me to melt into a little pool of water. Why're you looking at me like that?

STARK

I don't want him calling you Cleo. Who is he?

CLEO

(*Sitting*)

Oh, you! . . .

STARK

(*Angrily*)

I didn't call you Cleo till I knew you for weeks. Why should he?

CLEO

What's the matter with you anyway?

STARK

Nothing, Cleo.

CLEO

This whole thing has to end!

STARK

(*Staring at her*)

Does it?

CLEO

It can't go on like this. I'll go out with other men.

STARK

(*Crossing to her*)

No, you won't.

CLEO

I was thinking about you and your wife in Mr. Wax's office—

STARK

After the lecture we're going to the Planetarium—

CLEO

What did she say?

STARK

I don't care what she said.

CLEO

But I do—

STARK

After we visit the Planetarium—

CLEO

You don't think of me, don't care for me. . . .

188

STARK

We're going to leave early and have a cool supper. . . .

CLEO

Have a party by yourself!—

STARK

Listen to me. . . .

CLEO

I used to think you cared for me. . . .

STARK

But I do, Cleo. . . .

CLEO

Since when?

STARK

Since now. Tu amo, Cleo. . . . That means "I love you." You're right, darling. The stars are useless. I'll take you to a different place tonight.

CLEO

Where?

STARK

They won't know us from Adam there.

CLEO

But you don't love me.

189

STARK

Only you. Tonight we'll be together, Cleo. . . .
Alone, alone together. . . .

CLEO

I don't trust you.

STARK

You're more important to me than anything I
know. Cleo, dear. . . .

CLEO

What happened?

STARK

Nothing. I only know I love you, Cleo.

CLEO

(*After a pause, suddenly*)

Then hold me tight, Ben. Kiss me, love me—
kiss me till I can't be kissed no more. Hold me.
Don't let me be alone in the world, Ben. . . .
Don't let me be alone. . . . (STARK *moves to her
and they embrace passionately.*)

Curtain

ACT THREE

ACT THREE

PLACE: *The same.*
TIME: *Three weeks later, the end of August.*

BELLE *and* STARK *are present, he sitting motionlessly, a newspaper sprawled in his lap. She is sitting on the couch, looking over canceled checks.
There is a dead awful silence between them, each
one revolving in his own tight little world.*

*The office is only partly lighted. A spill of light
comes from the hallway left. Far off in the Hotel
Algiers a radio crooner is heard. A faint blue light
is burning in the operating room. The electric fan
hums busily. After a moment,* BELLE *looking up
obliquely,* STARK *goes to the fan, hoists its speed
and returns to his seat. Outside the waiting room
the air is hot and still, as before a storm.*

STARK

(*Finally*)

That fan must eat up juice a mile a minute. . . .
(*After further silence*) One of these days I'd like
to get air conditioning. Those small units aren't
expensive. . . .

BELLE

(*Suddenly*)

Why can't we drop this farce? Don't you owe me that much courtesy?

STARK

(*Stubbornly*)

Belle, I've told you the truth.

BELLE

You really stayed here to look over these vouchers?

STARK

I've told you so several times.

BELLE

You're looking for an eighteen-dollar error?

STARK

Since when do we sneeze at eighteen dollars?

BELLE

And that kept you here till nine at night?

STARK

(*Challengingly*)

Yes.

194

BELLE

(*Triumphantly*)

There's no mistake in these vouchers!

STARK

No? . . . Then *I've* made a mistake. But if I *didn't* check them over, you'd say I was careless. (*Shaking his head*) You can't win with a woman!

BELLE

Not my type.

STARK

I found that out years ago. (*Getting a sarcastically baleful glare from her*) I know, you've still got the girl on your mind.

BELLE

You're not waiting here for her?

STARK

No. (*He goes to the water cooler and drinks*)

BELLE

You don't think you owe me certain common courtesies?

STARK

And what may those be?

BELLE

The truth! The truth! The truth! (*Before* STARK *can answer, the office telephone rings.*)

STARK

(*Hurrying to the office door*)

I'll answer that.

BELLE

(*Blocking his way*)

No, I'll take it. (*They look at each other a moment.* STARK *finally steps to one side.* BELLE *picks up the telephone, looking out at* STARK.)

BELLE

Hello. . . . No, this isn't Miss Singer. Who is—? (BELLE *clips her words short. She proffers the phone to* STARK, *saying*) Your esteemed father-in-law. (STARK *takes the telephone nervously.*)

STARK

Yes, Poppa. . . . No, she isn't. . . . I don't know. . . . Tonight? . . . Well, don't come too late; I'll wait a half hour. Good-bye. (*He hangs up the telephone and comes into the waiting room*) Poppa's coming over. He wants to see me.

BELLE

What about?

STARK

He didn't say.

BELLE

You might have told him we're going home.

STARK

I'll call him back and tell him.

BELLE

But you don't want to go home.

STARK

(*Over-patient*)

I'll call him back and tell him.

BELLE

(*Insistently*)

Do you . . . ? (STARK *slowly turns and looks at her with a twisted face. Finally he says in a twisted voice.*)

STARK

No, Belle, I don't. That's a shack on the beach, and this is a shack. Don't be angry . . . it won't do us no good to quarrel again. I know you're my wife, but it's like we're enemies. We're like two exposed nerves!

BELLE

(*Bitterly*)

It's *my* fault!

STARK

(*Quietly*)

Much more mine. I don't know what happened. I thought about these things a lot these past few months. You expect many things from marriage, but I can't give them. I feel a moral obligation but I don't know what to do. These scenes go on. We're always worried . . . we're two machines counting up the petty cash. Something about me cheats you —I'm not the man to help you be the best woman it's in you to be. So your attitude's justified. I know I owe you a lot, Belle—

BELLE

(*Bitterly*)

Hallelujah!

STARK

(*Anger mounting despite himself*)

Now I realize I've had a guilty feeling for years. "Marriage is the only adventure open to the coward," a certain man says. He made a mistake; you have to be a hero to face the pains and disappointments. (*As she tries to speak*) No, let me finish. Because now I'm really guilty. . . . I mean with this girl—

BELLE

(*Quickly*)

That's enough!

STARK

I can't lie any more—

BELLE

That's enough! Do you hear me? Enough!

STARK

(*Insistently*)

I have to tell you—

BELLE

(*Jumping up*)

But you don't love her! You had an affair, all
right, but you don't *love* her! (STARK *sits, head in
hands.* BELLE *continues with fearful agitation*) The
girl was here all day. You were close together and
you fell into that thing. I can forget it, I can forget
it, Ben. I'm your wife. It doesn't involve our whole
relationship. We can have many happy years together. I'll do anything you want. We're young—
we have our life together in common, our ten
years. We can talk it out—we're civilized beings—
I'll never mention it. We'll both forget it! We need
each other, Ben. We . . . (BELLE *stands there,
wavering, a spout of water.* STARK *goes to her, embracing her. She is bloodless, stunned.*)

STARK

Belle, dear, dear, dear, dear. . . .

BELLE

(*Moving away and staring at him*)

It was only a thing of the moment, wasn't it? Wasn't it? Do you hear me—wasn't it?

STARK

(*Anything to blot out this pale ghost before him*)

Yes, yes! (*A pause, she wavers again, has to hold on to furniture to steady herself. Finally.*)

BELLE

(*Wildly*)

I'll wait for her. When is she coming back?

STARK

(*Frightened*)

I'll take you home, Belle. We'll go home. . . .

BELLE

When is she coming back here?

STARK

I don't know.

BELLE

(*Wildly*)

You don't know? Did you tell me you don't know? (*Sitting*) I'll sit and wait for her.

200

STARK

(*After a pause*)

Belle, you can't do that. . . . We'll talk about it tomorrow—we'll be more sensible—

BELLE

Do you love her?

STARK

(*Twisting*)

. . . It can't be settled in a minute, Belle.

BELLE

(*White to the lips*)

What can't be settled?

STARK

I don't know what. . . . I have a responsibility. . . .

BELLE

Your first responsibility's to me! You hear that?

STARK

I have to know what to do, Belle, and . . .

BELLE

To do? . . . You don't know what to do? You're in doubts? You have the slightest doubt?

STARK

(*Writhingly*)

I don't know what. . . .

BELLE

(*Instantly*)

Give me the key to the car!

STARK

I'll go down with you.

BELLE

Give me the key.

STARK

(*Giving her the key*)

It's across the street— I'll take you down. . . .

BELLE

Stay here.

STARK

Downstairs to the car. . . . (*She slaps him strongly across the face. He is silent.*)

BELLE

When you know what to do . . . I'll be at Milly Heitner's apartment. (*A blazing fury—but watery in the legs—she exits in silence.* STARK *stands in his place, literally shivering. Then he turns out a light. After a moment he sits, unable to stand. The newspaper has slipped to the floor; he picks it up and puts it in his lap. A knock sounds at the door—it is repeated—*STARK *pays no attention. Then the door knob is rattled.*)

FRENCHY

(*Without*)

Nobody home?

STARK

(*Clearing his throat*)

Who is it?

FRENCHY

Me, Doc—Frenchy. (*After* STARK *opens the door*) I knew I didn't see you leave. (STARK *has resumed his seat, newspaper in lap*) In the dark? Getting to be a poet in your old age, Doc?

STARK

(*Clearing his throat again*)

Cooler in the dark. . . .

FRENCHY

(*Sitting*)

The days are getting shorter . . . you notice that?

STARK

Yes. . . .

FRENCHY

It starts early.

STARK

What starts early?

FRENCHY

Night starts early. . . . I got a headache—some carbon knocking around in the dome. . . .

STARK

(*Abstracted*)

What?

FRENCHY

(*Giving him a shrewd glance*)

Who you sticking around for?

STARK

(*After a pause*)

. . . Cleo.

FRENCHY

Where is she?

STARK

(*After a pause*)

What? Out with Wax. . . .

FRENCHY

Again? (*Silence.*)

STARK

In a few weeks I'll be forty. . . .

FRENCHY

(*Giving him a sharp glance*)

Yeah? . . .

STARK

I feel like a boy. (*After a pause*) Did you ever wish to have some children?

FRENCHY

They break too easy. . . . (FRENCHY *waits for another question, which finally comes.*)

STARK

What do *you* get out of life?

FRENCHY

(*Blinking*)

I just woke up. I was reading a book before, and then I thought about it and then I fell asleep. What I get out of life?—Lemme think about it. Well . . . small change, I guess, but I like it. I tinker with my motors, the little boat and the jalopy. The jalopy cost me ninety bucks. Three times I took her apart and put it together again. Does General Motors himself get more fun?

STARK

But you're a man!—

FRENCHY

With all the accoutrements of man, I can't deny that.

STARK

Don't you want to get married?

FRENCHY

When it's time, Doc.

STARK

When you fall in love, you mean?

FRENCHY

(*With extreme seriousness*)

Love? Depends on what you mean by love. Love, for most people, is a curious sensation below the equator. Love—as they call it—is easy—even the rabbits do it! The girl I want . . . she'd have to be made in heaven. That's why I wait—

STARK

You're that good, you think?

FRENCHY

(*Correcting him*)

That *bad*, Doc! *She'll* have to be the good one. This is why: Love is a beginning, a jumping-off place. It's like what heat is at the forge—makes the metal easy to handle and shape. *But love and*

the grace to use it!—To develop, expand it, vari-
ate it!—Oh, dearie me, that's the problem, as the
poet said!

STARK

Yes, I see your point. . . .

FRENCHY

Who can do that today? Who's got time and
place for "love and the grace to use it"? Is it something apart, love? A good book you go to in a
spare hour? An entertainment? Christ, no! It's a
synthesis of good and bad, economics, work, play,
all contacts . . . it's not a Sunday suit for special occasions. That's why Broadway songs are
phony, Doc!—Love is no solution of life! Au con-
traire, as the Frenchman says—the opposite. You
have to bring a whole balanced normal life to love
if you want it to go!

STARK

Yes, I see your point.

FRENCHY

In this day of stresses I don't see much normal
life, myself included. The woman's not a wife.
She's the dependent of a salesman who can't make
sales and is ashamed to tell her so, of a federal
project worker . . . or a Cooper, a dentist . . .
the free exercise of love, I figure, gets harder every
day.

207

STARK

I see your point.

FRENCHY

We live in a nervous time. How can I marry? With what? . . . Unless the girl is with me, up to the minute on all these things. Otherwise they get a dirty deal, the girls.

STARK

(*Abstracted*)

Yes, I see. . . .

FRENCHY

You're not listening. . . .

STARK

(*Pale and strained*)

I heard most . . . of what you said.

FRENCHY

(*After a pause*)

I hope you excuse me, Doc; you and your wife woke me up before. . . .

STARK

Yes? . . .

FRENCHY

(*Starting hesitantly*)

Suppose . . . do you mind if I say this?

STARK

What? . . .

FRENCHY

(*Plunging in*)

Do you know what I'd ask myself? . . . What can I do for the girl, for Cleo? What will she be in ten years, with my help?

STARK

(*With a burning face*)

You talk as if a happy marriage isn't possible—

FRENCHY

No, I don't. But they're rare, like the dodo bird, mostly extinct. You know it yourself, Doc.

STARK

(*Suddenly bursting out*)

Frenchy, I love her, I love her! . . . I love that girl! I'm half out of my mind. I don't know what to do. (*Striding to the light switch*) Look at me. My face is so twisted. It feels twisted—is it twisted? . . .

FRENCHY

(*Quietly*)

Sit down, Doc.

STARK

I'm sick to my stomach. Where's my wife? Where did she go? Where's Cleo? She said she'd be back at seven. It's way past nine.

FRENCHY

No, sit down, Doc. Let's sit and talk. Let's be practical.

STARK

(*Out of control*)

Practical? Huh! What's practical about this slow exhaustion, this shame—not knowing what to do—I told my wife—I'm ready for the nut house—

FRENCHY

Leave the morals out. Sit down. Never mind the shame and guilt.

STARK

All my life I've been afraid to do something wrong and now I've done it.

FRENCHY

Leave the Scriptures out, Doc. Let's separate the problems. (STARK *stares at* FRENCHY *a moment, wags his head and sits, assisted by* FRENCHY.)

STARK

(*In a low voice, smiling faintly*)

I'm not sick. . . .

FRENCHY

(*After a pause*)

Leaving Scriptures out. . . . Do you want the girl or your wife? That's problem number one.

STARK

(*Mopping his head*)

I don't know where I stand. . . .

FRENCHY

Can you answer that tonight? (*The outer door knob is rattled from the outside.* FRENCHY *opens the door.* MR. PRINCE *steps in, rolled umbrella in hand, the handle a fancily carved dog's head of ivory.*)

PRINCE

Look, the gathering of the clans. What's here, a pinochle game? (*Sitting*) Where's Belle?—I heard her on the phone.

STARK

She went home.

FRENCHY

(*Looking from one to the other*)

And so will I. . . . (*Pointedly*) If no one minds? Doc?

STARK

I'll see you in the morning, Frenchy.

FRENCHY

That's a nice umbrella head you got there, Mr. Prince. Does he bite?

PRINCE

(Smiling smoothly)

A quiet dog always bites.

FRENCHY

(At the door)

Au revoir, gentry.

PRINCE

Gute nacht, mein Herr. (FRENCHY *exits.*)

STARK

Why so late, Poppa? It's nearly ten.

PRINCE

The logic is on your side. . . . (*Watching* STARK *wind his watch*) I seen Mrs. Heitner on the street today.

STARK

I hate that woman! (*Then masking his vehemence*) It's cooling off outside, isn't it?

PRINCE

Rain can be expected any minute. The good

Lord keeps a balance, dry and wet. . . . Yes, we face serious problems before us.

STARK

What problems?

PRINCE

I feel again the shudder of humility, Benny.

STARK

What? Why? (*Incredulously*) *What?*

PRINCE

The good Lord sees all, knows all. . . .

STARK

(*Impatiently*)

Don't be so circular, Poppa! What're you driving at?

PRINCE

Last night I fell asleep and dreamed the secret of the world. It is not good for Man to live alone. You hear?

STARK

I hear.

PRINCE

Where's Miss Cleo?

STARK

(*Briefly*)

Gone for the night.

PRINCE

You're not waiting for her?

STARK

No. Why?

PRINCE

(*Solemnly*)

Belle is getting suspicious.

STARK

(*Dry in the mouth*)

. . . Of what?

PRINCE

You have to get up like a morning glory to bamboozle me.

STARK

(*Angrily*)

What the hell are you trying to say?

PRINCE

(*Raising his voice*)

That a great thought occurred in my mind. To be frank, I like your taste.

STARK

I don't like these insinuations!

PRINCE

(*Suddenly standing up*)

Then come out in the open.

214

STARK

Poppa!—

PRINCE

Yes?

STARK

(*Wildly*)

Leave the office!

PRINCE

(*Solemnly*)

That's how you speak to King Midas? (*The two men stare at each other,* STARK *slowly turning away and getting himself in hand. Finally.*)

STARK

(*In a low voice*)

You're a wretched man, Mr. Prince.

PRINCE

(*Down to business*)

A desperate man, Dr. Benny. A man in love.

STARK

With whom?

PRINCE

Miss Cleo.

STARK

(*Incredulously*)

Miss? . . . Miss? . . .

PRINCE

Let us chew some brass tacks. You're having an affair with her. . . .

STARK

No!

PRINCE

I have experience—let *me* be the liar. (*Holding* STARK *with his eye*) It is my intention to renovate my life. Miss Cleo was elected on the first count: I want her in marriage.

STARK

Poppa!

PRINCE

She pleases my eye and ear—in every way a constant pleasure.

STARK

You must be out of your mind! Crazy! She won't have you!

PRINCE

(*The men standing face to face*)

You like to choke me? Do it . . . put your two hands on my old guzzle and squeeze! That's the only way you'll stop me!

STARK

(*After momentary consideration, shaking his head*)

No, you can't be sane!

PRINCE

Are you? What can you offer her? Did it ever enter your befuddled mind?

STARK

I won't discuss this! And leave the office!

PRINCE

She's coming back here tonight?

STARK

If I could only see your true face just once!

PRINCE

Is she?

STARK

(*Bitingly*)

Maybe!

PRINCE

Good!

STARK

(*Scornfully*)

You're very confident.

PRINCE

(*Quietly*)

I know human nature.

STARK

And you dare to think you'll buy that girl?
You're a damned smiling villain! Go home, get
out! (*A slow flush creeps up* PRINCE's *face. He
tries to hold back his anger, but it comes out
warmly.*)

PRINCE

Listen, a man in the fullness of his life speaks to
you. I didn't come here to make you unhappy. I
came here to make *myself happy!* You don't like
it—I can understand that. Circumstances insulted
me enough in my life. But *your* insults I don't
need! And I don't apologize to no man because I
try to take happiness by the throat! Remember,
Dr. Benny, I want what I want! There are seven
fundamental words in life, and one of these is
love, and I didn't have it! And another one is
love, and I don't have it! *And the third of these
is love, and I shall have it!* (*Beating the furniture
with his umbrella*) De corpso you think! I'm dead
and buried you think! I'll sit in the long winter
night with a shawl on my shoulders? Now you
see my face, Dr. Benny. Now you know your
father-in-law, that damned smiling villain! I'll
fight you to the last ditch—you'll get mowed
down like a train. I want that girl. I'll wait downstairs. When she returns I'll come right up, in five
minutes. I'll test *your* sanity!—*You,* you Nobel
prize winner! (*He stops, exhausted, wipes his face*

with a large silk handkerchief, does the same to the umbrella head and then slowly exits. STARK *stands motionlessly a moment, licking his lips nervously. He looks at his watch again, putting it to his ear. He hears a sound outside the window, rain. He goes to the window, right, putting his hand out to feel the rain. He puts the cool hand to his fevered face. With a handkerchief he mops his face and neck nervously. The door knob rattles;* STARK *immediately opens the door.* WILLY WAX *enters.*)

WAX

Hello, Dr. Stark-sky.

STARK

Oh, you. . . .

WAX

Mopping up your brain sweat?

STARK

It's hot enough. . . .

WAX

Raining out.

STARK

I can hear it.

WAX

(*Listening with over-intentness*)

That's right; you can hear it. Well, Stark-sky, your little Neon light spluttered right in my face.

That's a curious girl, that one. Was she ever an ice skater in the Olympics? She said she was.

STARK

(*Impatiently*)

Where is she?

WAX

Somewhere in the last century, where she belongs.

STARK

I beg your pardon?

WAX

I mean she's old-fashioned, romantic—she believes in love!

STARK

(*Coldly*)

I find her quite modern.

WAX

Because you're old-fashioned yourself.

STARK

Where is Miss Singer?

WAX

(*Chuckling*)

Sent her home. She thinks I'm a wolf.

STARK

So do I.

WAX

(*With a laugh*)

Got some business down my office. That's why I returned. (*He starts for the door.*)

STARK

Business with whom?

WAX

(*Suddenily dropping his mask of affability*)

None of your goddam business!

STARK

Is Miss Singer down there?

WAX

I told you she spluttered in my face, you idiot! Where do you think I got these scratches?

STARK

Where is she?

WAX

What's giving you cancer?

STARK

I want you to keep away from her.

WAX

You want *what?*

STARK

You have no interest in her, not the slightest. You have lots of girls, Wax—all you want and . . .

WAX

(*Jeeringly*)

This prosecuting-attorney role becomes you not.

STARK

(*Earnestly*)

Cleo's young, extremely naïve in some ways. You might warp her for life— (WAX *laughs*) Please, Wax, seriously— I must ask you to leave her alone. She's a mere mechanism to you, for a night—

WAX

Certainly, I'm a mechanical man in a mechanical era!

STARK

Please listen to me. . . .

WAX

You're making a clown of yourself. And secondly, since when does a stinker dentist, a prime pinhead, have the right to dictate the morals and manners of a Willy Wax!

STARK

You keep away from her!

WAX

(*Vehemently*)
You mind your goddam business!

STARK

Wax, for God's sake—!

WAX

Understand this for once and all: any white woman who pleases me— (STARK *abruptly plunges forward and seizes* WAX *by the throat.* WAX *is frightened out of his wits.*) Stark! Stop it! Stop . . . that! Are you . . . (STARK *releasing him*) nuts? . . . Are you nuts? (*Both men are breathing heavily, very pale, watching each other narrowly.* WAX, *a physical coward, immediately puts on a bold front*) That's how you act over a little pony who can't stand on her own legs? You're walking around in the shadow of the noose, Stark-sky. (*Making his clothing orderly*) Don't I know your type?—A bourgeois balcony climber —married, prates of purity—gives temperance lectures, but drinks and plays around—

STARK

Leave the office, please.

WAX

You're lucky I didn't eviscerate you!

STARK

Please, please. . . .

WAX

You want that girl yourself.

STARK

I'm asking you to—

WAX

(*Emphatically*)

No further commerce between us! (*Going to the door*) Years of dentistry have gone to your head. (*Before* WAX *can open the door* CLEO *has done so from the other side. She removes the key from the lock.* WAX *stiffly stands his ground.* CLEO *enters, soberly moving past him*) Well, it's not in my nature to hold a grudge. . . .

CLEO

(*Flashing on him*)

Mr. Wax, we don't want you around this office. You make love very small and dirty. I understand your type very well now. No man can take a bite out of me, like an apple and throw it away. Now go away, and we won't miss you.

WAX

(*Angrily*)

Yeah, I'm forming a Society for the Extermination of the Superfluous. You two are charter members! (WAX *exits, slamming the door behind him.* STARK *looks at* CLEO; *she is wearing a new colorful raincoat.*)

CLEO

It's raining like the devil.

STARK

I almost killed that man. . . . (*He looks down at his hands. Then he moves to the operating room and we see his back as he bends over the wash basin.*)

CLEO

(*Frightened*)

What're you doing?

STARK

Washing my hands.

CLEO

(*Glibly, making conversation*)

I went home for my new raincoat. That's why I'm late—aside from Mr. Wax. Don't you think this is a beautiful coat? (STARK *silently appears in the doorway, toweling his hands. Finally he flings the towel away and begins to prowl around the room.* CLEO *watches him, not knowing what to do or say. Finally* STARK *confronts her.*)

STARK

Cleo dear, we have to come to an understanding.

CLEO

(*Frightened*)

I think we do. . . .

STARK

(*After a pause*)

I feel so helpless . . . no judgment left. I don't know what I'm doing or saying. I almost want to cry. . . .

CLEO

Why, Ben? You have me—I didn't run away or do anything bad.

STARK

Do you love me very much?

CLEO

(*Simply*)

Yes.

STARK

Try to understand my problems, darling.

CLEO

At the moment the words "problem" and "darling" don't go together. You have to be honest with me, Ben. (*Taking his hand*) You must tell me what you're thinking. . . .

STARK

(*Hesitantly*)

Cleo, if I could . . . I don't know how to put it. . . . If . . .

CLEO

(*Trying to help him*)

What do you want to say? . . .

STARK

Help me. . . .

CLEO

How? (*Suddenly they embrace swiftly,* STARK *shaking all over.* PRINCE *now enters, finding them in this position. They do not see him until he speaks.* PRINCE *comes into the room.* CLEO *moves away from* STARK *and stares at* PRINCE.)

PRINCE

Excuse me—intrusion is not my purpose. (*To* STARK) Did you tell her? (*Receiving no answer from* STARK) I told Dr. Stark I love you—

CLEO

(*Looking from one to the other*)

You must be joking. . . .

PRINCE

No. . . . (*There is a silence during which the three persons look at one another.* CLEO *is annoyed and puzzled;* STARK *is sullen, nervous and angry, even a little hang-dog in attitude.* PRINCE *is determined and passionately desperate, but* CLEO'S *attitude adds a certain wariness to his demeanor. Finally*) I think we are ready for a preliminary analysis, as my friend Mr. Sugarman used to say.

STARK

(*With a curt laugh*)

Your aberration grows by the minute!

PRINCE

Look at him—the pebble sneers at the ocean!

CLEO

(*Warningly*)

Don't act high and mighty, Mr. Prince!

PRINCE

(*Warily*)

I come in all humility to propose marriage.

CLEO

You pick a bad time to joke.

PRINCE

No, Miss Cleo— Is this a comedian's face?

STARK

I think so.

PRINCE

(*Restraining his anger*)

I'm speaking to an intelligent young woman who'll understand my points.

CLEO

What points?

PRINCE

One by one, allow me to ask: why don't he (*pointing to* STARK) stand by your side? He's across the room, caving in. With what? Fear and worry. Why? He might lose you.

CLEO

(*Stoutly*)

He won't lose me!

PRINCE

Then *you* might lose *him*.

CLEO

(*Warningly*)

You'd better mind your business.

PRINCE

My love for you is my business. In the whole world I have no other business.

CLEO

Tell him to go home, Ben. It's your office—chase him out!

PRINCE

I admire your loyalty, Miss Cleo; but not Dr. Stark's. Give up a vain delusion—this man won't divorce his wife.

STARK

How can you . . . how do you dare! . . .

PRINCE

What, what? Tell us what, Benny! We want to hear your mind. What? (*But* STARK *doesn't know what to say and lapses into fuming knotted silence.* PRINCE *and* CLEO *both stare at him.*)

CLEO

(*To* PRINCE)

I don't want to hear another word from you. Do I have to slap your face to make you stop? Because you're an old man and I wouldn't like to

do that! And you can take your present back.
(*She tears off the coat and flings it at* PRINCE *who
tosses it to one side with the end of his umbrella*)
Ben, what're you waiting for? Why don't you say
something?

STARK

(*Writhing with indecision*)

Cleo. . . .

PRINCE

Give this girl a logical answer.

STARK

(*Bursting out*)

Cleo and I'll talk in private!

PRINCE

If I leave now, you'll give an answer?

CLEO

(*Turning on* STARK)

Are you going to let him go on like that?
(STARK'S *answer is again knotted writhing silence.*)

PRINCE

You are clay, Miss Cleo, on the way to great
womanhood. (CLEO *has been staring at* STARK,
*who is unable to meet her eyes. Now she turns
back to* PRINCE.)

CLEO

What did you say?

PRINCE

What can he offer you? He loves you—his
memoirs are written on his face. But I see a big
chapter heading: "No Divorce." Why not? Ten
years they're married. She runs his life like a credit
manager. They lost a child together . . . they're
attached underground by a hundred different
roots. But if he left her—as he knows—could he
leave his practice? Never! Then *you'd* be a credit
manager. . . . But why go on? He won't leave
her. That needs courage, strength, and he's not
strong.

CLEO

(*To* STARK)

Why don't you answer him? (*There is a momentary silence.* CLEO *is looking from one to the
other, realizing that* STARK *has no case.*)

PRINCE

(*Finally*)

My girl, I studied you like a scientist. I understand your needs.

CLEO

(*Not knowing what to do or say*)

What are they?

PRINCE

A man to help you learn and grow. A man of maturity and experience in everything—love, what to eat, where, what to wear and where to buy it—money to buy it—an eye turned out to the world! You need a man who is proud to serve you and has the means to do it. He knows how to speak to the head waiter and the captain on the ship. He don't look foolish before authority. He is a missionary in life with one mission, to serve and love you.

STARK

(*Laughing desperately*)

How absolute the knave is!

PRINCE

Now let us come down to terra firma. You're a brilliant girl. . . . I'm old enough to be your father.

CLEO

Well?

PRINCE

But notice! Every president of this great country is my age. Because this is the time he's at his best. . . . He has learned how to serve. And there is a simple worldly consideration—it has its importance. In twenty years you'll still be young, a beautiful woman of the world. Cremate me, burn me up and throw me away, and what have you

233

got? A fortune! And so you go, a great woman, scattering good as you go. . . .

CLEO

(*After a pause*)

What do you say, Ben? (*After waiting*) Don't stand there like a dead man. . . .

PRINCE

What can he say? He's as mixed up as the twentieth century!

STARK

(*Turning wrathfully on* PRINCE)

You come here with this lust!

CLEO

(*Shaking* STARK *by the arm*)

Don't fight with him. Talk to *me*, Ben.

PRINCE

Time is of the essence.

CLEO

(*Almost crying*)

Don't discuss him, Ben. Tell me what *our* plans are. What'll you do with me?

STARK

Cleo, I can't talk now. . . . This man standing here . . .

CLEO

No, you have to tell me now. Where do I stand? . . .

STARK

(*Evasively*)

Stand? . . .

PRINCE

(*Harshly*)

In short, will you leave your wife? (STARK *is silent, unable to make an answer.* CLEO *looks at him appealingly.* PRINCE *stands in the background, unwilling to provoke* CLEO's *wrath.*)

CLEO

What do you say, Ben . . . ?

STARK

(*Lost*)

Nothing. . . . I can't say . . . Nothing. . . .

CLEO

You'll let me go away? (*She gets no reply from him. Half stunned, she seats herself. Finally.*)

CLEO

I'd like to hold my breath and die.

PRINCE

(*Softly*)

He'd let you do that, too.

STARK

(*To* PRINCE)

You're a dog, the lowest dog I ever met! (*To* CLEO) Do you know what this man is trying to do?

CLEO

(*Crushed*)

I don't care.

STARK

(*Gently*)

Listen, Cleo . . . think. What can I give you? All I can offer you is a second-hand life, dedicated to trifles and troubles . . . and they go on forever. This isn't self-justification . . . but facts are stubborn things, Cleo; I've wrestled with myself for weeks. This is how it must end. (*His voice trembling*) Try to understand . . . I can't say more. . . . (*He turns away. There is a momentary silence, which is broken by* PRINCE.)

PRINCE

(*Approaching her from the other side*)

And I offer you a vitalizing relationship: a father, counselor, lover, a friend!

CLEO

(*Wearily*)

Why don't you stop it, Mr. Prince?

PRINCE

Because I mean it.

CLEO

I see you mean it. But you forget one thing—
I don't love you.

PRINCE

(*Insistently*)

Put yourself in my hands. . . .

CLEO

(*Wanly*)

I think I have to leave now.

PRINCE

Wear this . . . it's wet outside. (PRINCE *picks up the raincoat and spreads it for her.*)

CLEO

(*Smiling faintly*)

Would it make you happy if I kept it? (*He nods soberly. She goes to him and slips into the coat. Suddenly, from behind, he grips her two arms.*)

PRINCE

Miss Cleo, believe me, life is lonely, life is empty. Love isn't everything. A dear true friend is more than love—the serge outlasts the silk. Give me a chance. I know your needs. I *love* your needs. . . . What do you have to lose?

237

CLEO

(*Immobile*)

Everything that's me.

PRINCE

What is you? You haven't arrived yet. You're only on the way to being you.

CLEO

I don't want you, Mr. Prince. I'm sorry.

PRINCE

(*Passionately*)

You can't refuse me! What do you want?

CLEO

I don't know. . . .

PRINCE

(*As above*)

By what you don't know, you can't live! You'll never get what you're looking for! You want a life like Heifetz's music—up from the roots, perfect, clean, every note in place. But that, my girl, is music!

CLEO

I'm looking for love. . . .

238

PRINCE

From a book of stories!

CLEO

Don't say that. I know what's real. (*Of* STARK)
Is his love real?

PRINCE

But *mine!* . . .

CLEO

It's real for *you.* If I can't find love here, I'll
find it there.

PRINCE

(*Insistently*)

Where?

CLEO

Somewhere. . . . How can I tell you what I
mean? . . .

PRINCE

You'll go down the road alone—like Charlie
Chaplin?

CLEO

(*To both men*)

Yes, if there's roads, I'll take them. I'll go up
all those roads till I find what I want. I want a
love that uses me, that needs me. Don't you think
there's a world of joyful men and women? Must
all men live afraid to laugh and sing? Can't we
sing at work and love our work? It's getting late
to play at life; I want to *live* it. Something has to

feel real for me, more than both of you. You see? I don't ask for much. . . .

PRINCE

She's an artist.

CLEO

I'm a girl, and I want to be a woman, and the man I love must help me be a woman! Ben isn't free. He's a citizen of another country. And you, Mr. Prince, don't let me hurt your feelings; you've lived your life. I think you're good, but you're too old for me. And Mr. Wax, his type loves himself. None of you can give me what I'm looking for: a whole full world, with all the trimmings! (*There is a silence.* PRINCE *sees he is licked. Finally he sighs and says softly.*)

PRINCE

Silence is better than rubies. . . .

CLEO

Experience gives more confidence, you know. I have more confidence than when I came here. Button my coat, Ben.

STARK

(*Coming right to her*)

Yes. . . . (*He quickly buttons the front of her coat with fumbling nervous hands. Then suddenly*

he embraces her strongly, tears in his eyes) How
your heart beats, Cleo . . . how it beats. . . .

CLEO
(*Finally, as they separate*)

I understand you, Ben. . . . Good night.
(STARK *is silent.* PRINCE *shakes his head and says.*)

PRINCE

I'll drive you home.

CLEO

No, I'll go alone. Don't follow me—stay here.
Count a hundred till I'm gone. . . .

PRINCE

Good-bye, Miss Cleo.

CLEO
(*As they gravely shake hands*)

Good-bye, Mr. Prince. If you close your eyes,
you'd never know I'd been here. Count a hundred—

PRINCE
(*Closing his eyes*)

One, two, three . . . four, five . . . (CLEO
has left the room. PRINCE *slowly opens his eyes*)
. . . fifteen, thirty-seven, eighty-nine . . . (*Then*

241

in a whisper) one hundred. . . . Lebewohl! I'm a judge of human nature. She means it; why don't we walk with shut eyes around in the world? . . . (*Looking at his watch*) It's very late. . . .

STARK

(*Who has been listening intently*)

There! . . . The elevator took her down. . . .

PRINCE

Yes, you love her. But now, my iceberg boy, we both have disappeared.

STARK

(*Tremblingly*)

I don't believe that. This isn't disappearance, when you're living, feeling what you never felt before. . . .

PRINCE

(*Heavily*)

Yes. . . .

STARK

(*Eyes flooding with tears*)

I insist this is a beginning. Do you hear?—I insist.

PRINCE

I hear. . . . (*He slowly moves to the door*) My mind is blank. Next week I'll buy myself a dog. . . .

STARK

You going home, Poppa?

PRINCE

It's Labor Day on Monday. In the morning I'm going to the mountains. I excuse you for the names you called me . . . as you excuse me.

STARK

Yes. . . .

PRINCE

(*Smiling faintly*)

You'll permit me to come around and disturb you, as usual. Good-bye, Benny.

STARK

Good-bye, Poppa. (*They smile at each other.* PRINCE *goes to the door.*)

PRINCE

(*At the door*)

Go home, to my daughter. . . .

STARK

(*Slowly rises from his seat; calls* PRINCE *back*)

Poppa, wait a minute. . . . (*Gropingly*) For years I sat here, taking things for granted, my wife, everything. Then just for an hour my life was in a spotlight. . . . I saw myself clearly, realized who and what I was. Isn't that a beginning? Isn't it? . . .

PRINCE

Yes. . . .

STARK

And this is strange! . . . For the first time in years I don't feel guilty. . . . But I'll never take things for granted again. You see? Do you see, Poppa?

PRINCE

Go home, Benny. . . . (*He turns out the lamp.*)

STARK

(*Turning out the other lamp*)

Yes, I, who sat here in this prison-office, closed off from the world . . . for the first time in years I looked out on the world and saw things as they really are. . . .

PRINCE

(*Wearily*)

It's getting late. . . .

STARK

(*Almost laughing*)

Sonofagun! . . . What I don't know would fill a book! (PRINCE *exits heavily.* STARK *turns out*

244

the last light, then exits, closing the door behind him. The room is dark, except for red neon lights of the Hotel Algiers and a spill of light from the hall.)

Slow curtain